D0069765

WORLD'S GREATEST WEIGHT LOSS

THE TRUTH THAT DIET GURUS DON'T WANT YOU TO KNOW

BRIAN QUEBBEMANN, M.D.

CONTENTS

"It's not so much that a person wins, but that they refuse to lose that results in success" - Brian Quebbemann, M.D.

SECTION 1:

WHY YOU WANT TO LOSE WEIGHT

WHY YOU ARE HOLDING THIS BOOK

If you are thumbing through this book in a bookstore or browsing through it online, there is probably one main reason: Whatever you have done in the past to gain control over your weight has not worked. Maybe it worked for a while, but nothing you have tried resulted in long-term success.

That is why I wrote this book.

The people who walk in my door have accepted the fact that they've failed, they've tried hard and still failed. The fact that they've tried and failed does not represent weakness, it shows strength. To admit that they need help and then to go out and get it takes a lot of strength. Giving up, now *that's* weakness.

"I now celebrate November 26th each year. This was my surgery date. I celebrate this day as much as my actual birthday because this is when I began my new life! Today I have lost over half my body weight. I weigh 175 pounds and have never been happier. About four months after my surgery I discovered how it felt to walk to the top of the stairs without losing my breath. By six months after surgery I was trying things that I never would have even dreamed of in my old life. I had taken up surfing, playing tennis and running. I ran my first 5K September of 2008! I run races regularly now. My life has turned around."

Michelle G.
Payroll Manager

My patients are the strong ones, no question. They aren't like all the other obese people that come out, try another diet in a long line-up of repeated diets, fail, and then surrender to the claim that it doesn't matter. My patients aren't willing to pretend it doesn't matter. They are the ones determined to go out and find a better answer, a different strategy.

You aren't the only one responsible for your excess weight. The fast food industry, our stressful society, the lousy diet advice you've been given…all of it has contributed to your perpetual weight-loss failure. The biggest factor might be the fact that almost nobody knows much about obesity and they know even less about weight loss.

"Having a career that emphasizes health and physical fitness, you would think I would naturally be motivated to stay in shape. I have always been physically active, playing sports, working out at the gym, etc. So it was easy for me to eat what I wanted and gain weight, then lose it when I needed to. I lost weight going from one diet to another, always gaining more weight after losing weight because I never made permanent lifestyle changes.

"My string of luck ended after turning 40. I had to have back surgery for two blown discs, and it took a long time to get back to normal activities. I eventually transferred to an office assignment and my weight *really* ballooned. Becoming a Type II diabetic really didn't motivate me to keep in shape, because I knew I had always been able to lose weight any time I wanted to. But by my late forties, I couldn't motivate myself to stay with any diet long enough to get back into shape.

"I felt gastric bypass would give me the best chance to get control of my health once and for all."

Edward G.
Fire Chief, Retired

"My wife and I were also planning on having a baby and I wanted to be an active father rather than one just sitting on the sidelines. I was 310 pounds, unhappy and I didn't want to end up with diabetes and other health problems. I wanted to be around to see my kids grow up and go to college and be able to participate in their activities."

Arran Nathaniel A.
Insurance Broker

The sad reality is, most books about dieting will doom you to failure. They give you rules to follow that, once broken, make you feel like a cheater. That's not what I do in my clinic and that's not the purpose of this book. My goal is to make you aware of the simple fact that *people who stay in shape don't follow a lifestyle they **hate*** *in order to be thin. Rather, people who stay in shape have found a lifestyle that they **enjoy** that keeps them fit.*

Millions of people buy self-help books on dieting and weight loss, and try to follow magic formulas that rarely, if ever, turn out to be magic. And when readers can't follow the rules listed in the book, they blame themselves and say, "I've failed."

But they don't give up. They move on to the next weight-loss formula and the result is the same. They are caught in a vicious cycle: Fight to stick with it, fail, frustrate, get fed up, get fatter, find another formula, and repeat, on and on...

Some of the "experts" writing such books are people who have lost weight successfully and then promote their habits as the answers for everyone with a weight problem. Other weight-loss experts are *researchers* who have studied the science of food, obesity and disease, and have come up with a set of rules based on *lab experiments*. Still others explain how certain foods prevent disease.

The problem is that these habits, answers and rules rarely take into consideration how people really want to live. They impose a set of rules and requirements that, by their design, are outside most people's needs and habits. This is a formula for failure.

As a physician who has dedicated my professional career to weight control, it's clear to me that many of the diet formulas offered are painfully confusing and ultimately inadequate. The longer I practice, the more convinced I become that diet *alone* is never the answer to lasting weight loss. Nor are medications or even surgery. After over 20 years helping people control their weight, I've seen what permanent weight loss looks like, and every time I see it the successful patient has developed a deep understanding of "Why." They understand and embrace the fact that there is more to it than diet alone. Permanent weight loss requires this understanding, and that's the main reason so many diet programs fail.

Acknowledging results, good or bad, rather than denying them, is the smart thing to do. If you're reading this book you've already figured that out. You know you need to find a different strategy and you're actively looking for one. What I'm here to tell you is that the best option for you might be surgery.

This book is for people who have found that non-surgical methods are not working, and are looking for a better alternative. Weight-loss surgery is not the answer for everyone and it's certainly not the only solution. It takes effort, involves some risks, and is definitely not the easy way out. But, for those struggling with obesity and not finding success using other methods, surgery may be your best answer.

Before you continue reading this book, there is one scientifically supported fact that I want you to know. At the time of writing this book, bariatric surgery is the single most successful method for obese people to achieve long-term weight loss. Bariatric surgery routinely succeeds when all other methods have failed, making it truly the world's greatest weight loss method available.

"It's not so much that a person wins, but that they refuse to lose that results in success." - **Brian Quebbemann, M.D.**

YOU ARE NOT TO BLAME

Billions of people are overweight or obese, and the reasons are many:

- Our cultures glorify food.

- Marketing has made necessities out of non-essential snacks.
- Most social gatherings revolve around eating.
- We are eating more low-nutrition, high-fat foods.
- Highly processed foods often contain empty calories in the form of sugar.
- Fewer and fewer people exercise on a regular basis.
- Most diets are ineffective at permanent weight loss.

In short, the odds are stacked against anyone living in the modern world who wants to stay fit.

"I'd had firsthand experience with weight regain after massive weight loss. Since adolescence, I'd lost 100 pounds or more on at least three occasions, through conventional diet and exercise only to start regaining the weight in a year or less, and to add insult to injury, the weight regain was always more than the original weight lost. In 1994 I went from 375 pounds to 220 pounds for a 155-pound weight loss. By the year 2000, I'd regained all the lost weight, and instead of weighing 375, now I weighed 400 pounds.

"With my personal history of weight loss and weight regain, I believe my skepticism of weight loss surgery being a permanent solution was reasonable. Nevertheless, at this juncture in my life I felt absolutely trapped and cornered!!! Personally, I felt defeated in the battle of weight, and was quite accepting of my fate."

Doug S.
Business Owner

"Why do I have a weight problem whenever I'm not on a diet?" In short, you have a weight problem for the same reason most of America has a weight problem. We all share a genetic predisposition to gain weight when we are sedentary and overeat. And there are numerous factors that play into why we overeat. One factor that you may or may not have considered is that *it's good for business*.

I have a patient, a successful investor, who bought a chain of 7-Eleven stores. One day, during a visit to my clinic, he said "I know why we're all fat." As a weight-loss expert I was a bit weary of hearing so many simple answers to this complicated problem, but he was a particularly intelligent guy, so I listened.

"OK, tell me why we're all fat," I responded.

He said, "Do you know what I want to sell you when you come into one of my 7-Elevens?"

I told him I had no idea.

"Slurpees," he said. He continued that every dollar you pay for a cup of the frozen, flavored sugar water represents a profit of 98 cents to him. "You buy Slurpees, I get rich." It was his best profit margin, but it was bad news for everyone who buys them.

I never checked the facts on this, but the point is, we are inundated with cheap sugars and fats virtually everywhere we turn. We eat fast food and snacks that aren't good for us and make us fat because they're cheap, quick, and promoted intensely—simply because they are so profitable. Never mind that a person can eat much healthier food for the same price or less. We usually take the convenient way out while "Mr. 7-Eleven" laughs all the way to the bank.

But obesity is no laughing matter. When we gain weight, we feel less comfortable exercising and our physical activity plummets.

As our muscle tone decreases, weaker muscles make us even less likely to engage in physical activity, leading to even more weight gain and obesity.

HOW WE GOT HERE

Understand that our genetic make-up, after 200,000 years of human existence, has not suddenly changed over the past 50. We are pretty much the same people that were alive in the 1950s, in 1900, in 1800 and further back. And, there were very few obese people living during those years. So, what has changed?

What has changed is our society: we are no longer required to put in much effort to obtain food, there is a huge abundance of high-calorie, low-quality food, and much of that is engineered to stimulate our natural craving for salt and fat. Our lives are, for the most part, so sedentary that many of us don't even develop the muscles we are genetically programmed to build. And, there are numerous ways to entertain ourselves that don't involve physical activity. The fact is, we've created the culture of the blob; we can just sit there and have stimulating images delivered in front of us, so we "interact" in a virtual space that exists only in our imagination. If it weren't for our need to care for basic bodily functions like cleaning ourselves, we could, conceivably, just sit for our entire lives, and eat, and be stimulated by toys, games and virtual reality until we expired.

The logical extension of this is that we eventually create a society where we live in our minds, and interact with each other through portals that channel our thoughts—we don't even have to move—and the sole purpose of our bodies is to support our minds.

Maybe we would eventually not even need our body! Wouldn't all this be wonderful!

Of course, we wouldn't ever really go hiking, we wouldn't really play basketball or soccer, there would be no Olympics and even sex would simply be something that we dreamed about but never really did. Some people may think that this is utopia, but for the time being we are stuck with our bodies, we need them, and so we need to take care of them, like a car or a bicycle. Maybe someday the human race, such as it is then, will not need bodies. Enjoying nature and the natural world will not be necessary, or even possible. We will be content to be blobs. Maybe this day will come. But until then we need our bodies. And, I'm extremely happy that I will not be alive if that type of world ever becomes our reality.

My guess is that humankind will become extinct long before this dream state comes to pass. Maybe a life-form such as Human Amoebas will develop. It's a thought. Nevertheless, I'm not ready to become a human amoeba yet. I like my body and the things it can do. I enjoy being able to have real fun in a real world and experience the real beauty that Mother Nature has provided. So, for now, I am happy and willing to develop the habits that allow me to remain healthy so that I can participate in life.

We are all obviously creatures of habit. If I were to paint the bottoms of your feet with black ink when you went grocery shopping, so that you would leave tracks throughout the grocery store, I would have a good idea of where you walked and what you bought. If I checked the patterns of your tracks after ten grocery shopping trips, I would find that you go to the same places, and buy the same things, almost every time. Even if I bundled you up and flew you to a different state where the grocery store had a different floor plan, your tracks would show me that you bought the same foods you typically purchased back home.

This is your grocery pattern, your eating pattern. This way of eating is your dietary habit. If you are going to take in different amounts of calories, you are going to have to change your habits. In other words, you are going to have to go to different places in the store, try different foods, and develop new habits.

If your dietary goal after any weight-loss program, surgical or otherwise (see my upcoming book on non-surgical weight loss, "The N.E.W. Program"), is to get back to a comfortable, convenient and familiar eating pattern (like the one that caused you to be overweight in the first place), you can do it, and guess what, you'll eventually be the same weight you were before.

However, after surgery you have an amazing amount of leverage to *change* your eating pattern. And this leverage is the difference between surgical weight loss and non-surgical weight loss. But you still have to use the leverage and change your habits.

If you're suddenly thinking, "But, I like the way I eat," you need to understand that there are many other eating patterns that would satisfy you completely and leave you happy and at a healthy weight. Do not believe that, somehow, any single dietary regimen is *the only one* compatible with your life. If that's the case, put this book down now and forget about permanent weight loss.

I can line up 20 people that are your same gender, your height, your bone and muscle structure, and your age, that are living at the weight you *wish* you were at. These twenty people don't stay at that weight because they are always dieting. If you ask them why they eat the way they do they'll look at you like you're a bit slow-minded and say, "Because I like it." Not only that, but these

20 people all have different eating patterns. So, here are 20 eating patterns that could work for you.

And, if you tell me that you don't like any of those eating patterns, I will find 20 *more* people that meet the same criteria, and they will have an *additional* 20 different eating patterns, so now you have 40 to choose from. So, pick one. On the other hand, if you find your own eating pattern, that's enjoyable and leaves you at a healthy weight, then you will become number 41 in this list of people. Simple.

WILLPOWER IS *NOT* THE ISSUE

Every week I'm faced with patients who tell me they are considering surgery because they "have no willpower." The shocking thing is, they believe this! Among this group are entrepreneurs who are running their third successful corporation, men that have four successful and happy grown children, and women that are active in civic groups and volunteer helping others. It's sad when patients willing to consider surgery, a very demanding step towards making a lifestyle change look down, embarrassed, and tell me, "I'm here because I have no willpower." And I'm there thinking "Willpower is definitely not your problem."

These people have become convinced that they have no willpower and this can be a problem going forward.

"A former competitive athlete, I was very self-conscious about my weight. My feet hurt and my clothes looked awful on me, so now, rather than play sports, I avoided outdoor activities. It was miserable having to sit alone and watch my kids swim, ski, play, go to the beach...and I just sat there. I was obsessed with guilt about being fat, I shouldn't have eaten that, what will I eat next, when can I eat next, but I shouldn't eat, on and on. That thought process playing over and over in my head was paralyzing."

Sandra L., R.N.
Director of Clinical Appeals

Blaming yourself is not helpful, at all. The fact is, you tried dieting and that failed; now you simply need a better strategy. In order to be successful with weight-loss surgery you need to *stop criticizing yourself*. Focus instead on what you are going to do now to make this a success.

"Dream, and chase those dreams. Too many people aren't brave enough to do the first, and don't have the strength to do the second." - Brian Quebbemann, M.D.

WE CAN DO BETTER THAN DIETING

Obesity is now an epidemic in America and in every modern country in the world. But, until the publication of this book, the prevailing "solution" to obesity has been something I liken to torture: forcing sane, normal people to continuously suffer as they try to follow one "scientifically derived" formula for a healthy weight after another. This is *traditional* dieting, which I refer to as a "Personal Persecution Program."

Simple diet and exercise programs may work for some people, but most often, Personal Persecution Programs are rigid "solutions" that are hard to follow long term. Worse, they don't have to make sense for people to try them. Since they aren't illegal to sell, they will always be dangled out there to lure desperate people into trying the same type of thing over and over again. But if you want an intelligent solution that may lead to permanent success, then you deserve something more.

The truth is that using surgery to help get the weight off once and for all is far better statistically, in terms of your health, than continuously carrying around all that extra fat. Medical research has proven this time and again. But, as I explain in this book, surgery is *not* the easy way out. Surgery is simply the best solution for many people *if it is used effectively.*

Weight-loss programs are often too narrow in their focus to be successful. Diet books talk only about food and eating habits. Exercise gurus focus only on "burning off the calories." Even bariatric surgery will fail if the surgeon focuses only on which surgical technique to use and not enough on addressing the *real* reason many people struggle to get rid of their obesity in the first place. The key to their struggle becomes apparent when you look at the habits of people who are successful.

I work in the field of obesity and excess weight professionally, but I've also been around athletes my entire life. One thing that has always been apparent to me is that nobody with lifelong fitness maintains their fit weight by constant dieting. I've observed that people who maintain a healthy weight for most of their lives do so *because they love doing what they have to do to maintain that healthy weight.*

This understanding is a fundamental principle of this book: understand *why* people who succeed at maintaining a lifelong healthy weight do so and apply this "why" to people who undergo surgery for obesity.

CHRONIC DIETING WILL RUIN YOUR LIFE

That's no surprise to anyone who has been overweight and on diets for a long time. It's the Yo-Yo Syndrome, and it goes like this: You are sure being overweight is ruining your life, so you try yet another diet. You lose a lot of weight. You stick with it for a while, but then you "lose willpower." You quit the diet, regain the weight and soon you're heavier than you were before. The cycle repeats.

Over time, you become a chronic dieter. You know you're overweight but, despite all the dieting, you don't have the "willpower" to stay on a diet forever. You are convinced the excess weight is ruining your life. Maybe your excess weight is affecting your health. But what really makes you miserable is thinking that, because of the extra weight, you'll be on a diet for the rest of your life.

THE DIETING MYTH

If you think dieting will keep you thin, take it from me: You're wrong. In my experience, *the longer you remain fixated on dieting, the fatter you will become.*

Almost all of my patients admit to trying many of the latest fad diets. My question is always the same: "How's it working for you?" The response is often a slightly embarrassed, somewhat defeated chuckle. I tell my surgical weight-loss patients to go home, put all their diet books into a box, and have it delivered to a skinny enemy, because if that person reads them and gets fixated on the goofy advice, he or she will eventually gain weight, too.

What the diet industry doesn't want you to know is that their diets will make you miserable. They are counting on you being unwilling to stay miserable forever in order to control your weight. So, you'll keep falling off their diet, regaining weight, and then you'll be back. They are selling the idea that you want nothing more than to be thin, and the way to be thin is by sticking to their diet.

That is what makes me call most diets a Personal Persecution Program. They make people miserable.

"As a child I never had any kind of a weight problem. It was not until I had my first child, 12 years ago, that I suddenly started packing on the pounds. Three children and 100+ pounds later I was frustrated, exhausted, and scared. I had tried everything to lose weight. You name the diet, pill, or program, and I tried it. I used to pray for a thyroid problem as it would be so much easier than facing the rest of my life as an obese adult."

Pia P.
Mother

THE EXERCISE MYTH

People sometimes think that exercise alone will result in substantial, permanent weight loss. Well, there are a lot of ways to explain why this is ridiculous. One way is to acknowledge that we can eat enough calories and nutrition in about 30 minutes to sustain us throughout the day, day after day, for our entire life. This means that we can eat enough in half an hour to sustain an active healthy life throughout a 24-hour day. No matter how hard we exercise, or how hard we work, we can consume more than enough calories in 30 minutes to *prevent* weight loss! Wow!

This is truly amazing. We humans have survived in part because we are such phenomenal eaters. We can eat so much in such a short time that, if food is available, it's impossible for us to starve! Not only are we phenomenal eaters, we love to eat. We are the descendants of the best food foragers and eaters in human history.

Now, take this gene pool and give it pizza delivery, fast food and no need to get off our lazy asses in order to survive, and we wonder why we are all becoming so fat. Even if we aren't lazy, and we exercise regularly, we can eat far more calories than the exercise will ever "burn off." Now, when you ask why an hour a day of exercise is not enough to overcome bad eating habits, you have your answer. The excess calories you can consume will destroy you. Forget about nuclear war; the real weapons of mass destruction are fast food, highly processed carbs, and high-fructose corn syrup!

WHAT'S WRONG WITH TRYING A WEIGHT-LOSS DIET?

The answer is "nothing." We just reviewed that healthy eating is critical, so why not try a diet?

Trying non-surgical weight-loss methods is not at all a bad idea, and trying a diet and exercise program is not a mistake. In fact, I highly recommend it as an initial step. But almost all severely obese people have too much to overcome, and will fail over and over again using those methods. You know this, and that's the reason you are reading this book.

It amazes me when I read popular weight-loss books and find, at the very beginning, an admission by the author that he or she does NOT specialize in weight control. Then, they go on to present a "foolproof formula." Even more amazing is that millions of people buy those books and try to follow the magic formulas that rarely, if ever, turn out to be magic. Then, after the foolproof formula doesn't work, the readers go on to the next popular weight-loss formula and the result is the same.

As a physician who has dedicated my professional career to weight control, it's clear to me that most formulas are painfully confusing and often inadequate. The longer I practice, the more convinced I become that simple diets are never the complete answer to lasting weight loss. It runs far deeper than that.

IGNORE BAD ADVICE FROM THE BENEVOLENT UNINFORMED

I see it in my practice all the time: well-intended advisors who think that losing weight is just a matter of "sheer will."

Take Kim. I happened to be dating Kim's roommate at the time and she had referred Kim to me. Kim was 200 pounds overweight and had a BMI greater than 60. Kim attended an appointment in my clinic and decided to proceed with bariatric surgery. Two weeks prior to her surgery, I happened to be out and about with my girlfriend and we stopped by at her apartment. Kim's mother was visiting from out of town. After we were introduced her mother told me, "I think Kim can do this on her own. She just needs to eat healthy and exercise." Remember, this comment was just a couple of weeks before Kim's already scheduled surgery.

I was taken aback, and then I got really pissed off. Kim needed support, not more negativity and criticism. I asked her mom if that's the same advice she'd been giving Kim for decades and Mom said, "Of course." Then I pointed out how smart Kim was, and how she was successful at her job despite her weight, and that she was so determined to get the weight off that she was preparing for surgery. I said that besides the fact that her mother's advice showed profound ignorance about the physiology of severe obesity, if her advice had been worthwhile, Kim wouldn't be so obese today. I then added, sarcastically, that maybe Kim was just stupid, or maybe she didn't try hard enough during the past two decades. But, I said, in my opinion, Kim had tried desperately for years and now she had decided to use surgery as a way to succeed, and I thought that showed intelligence and strength.

I was really quite upset at Kim's mom in the face of this eleventh-hour sabotage. This was not what Kim needed, and since she was my patient, I was going to stand up for her, period!

Everyone was quiet. Then, Mom acquiesced, grudgingly. Kim went on, had her surgery—with her mother's support—and was quite successful.

A HISTORY OF BAD IDEAS WITH GOOD INTENTIONS

Before we move on to the right way to achieve your best results from bariatric surgery, a little medical history might provide some useful perspective. In the mid-1900s there used to be a surgery that completely prevented people from eating normally. It was used on obese people, mostly younger people, and it was called jaw wiring. The unfortunate victims of these horrific procedures would be forced to live on liquids sucked through a straw in order to stay alive. They wouldn't get the satisfaction of chewing, their jaw would hurt because it was wired closed in one position for months, and everyone around them could eat normally…but they could not. This horrible treatment was, in my opinion, a form of torture, and of course it achieved nothing good.

Jaw wiring is a dark chapter in the history of medicine but, despite the fact that nobody with any sense of humanity would ever recommend something like this, I've been asked by some doctors, "Why do you do what you do? Why don't you just wire fat people's jaws shut?" Usually this stupid question is accompanied by an equally stupid chuckle. Well, suffice it to say that bariatric surgery is not like this. It does not force you into a rigid, restricted, unnatural eating pattern.

Modern bariatric surgery helps you develop new eating habits that allow you to control your weight permanently. Modern bariatric surgery helps you develop constructive habits, but you still have a choice in how you design them. That's how bariatric surgery works.

ANOTHER SHORT BUT TRUE STORY FROM DR. Q

A patient recently informed me that a local bariatric surgeon instructs all his patients to avoid all natural carbohydrates, including fruit and vegetables, after surgery until they've lost 75% of their excess body weight. I asked this patient what that surgeon allowed his patients to eat and she responded, "meat, fish, chicken and protein drinks." This patient had attended several support groups and said, "Everyone sits around in the support group talking about how they crave salads, or an apple."

I was astounded. First, I've never had a patient tell me, "Doc, I'm obese because I eat too many apples." Second, the average bariatric surgery patient loses less than 75% of excess weight, so these people are essentially being told that they can't eat fresh fruit and fresh vegetables for the rest of their lives. Third, how can patients develop new eating patterns if their entire period of weight loss involves surviving on meat and medical meal replacements?

I asked this patient whether the program seemed to be working and she told me, "No. The only thing everyone talks about at support groups is how they crave crunchy foods, and how they cheat by snacking on chips and stuff." This is a great example of how pushing rigid, ridiculous diet rules on patients results in them falling into dysfunctional eating habits, rather than learning how to make reasonable diet choices for themselves.

Bariatric surgery is not intended to permanently force people to eat a certain way. True, you won't be able to gobble food down, but other than that, most people eat quite normally over time. Bariatric surgery also doesn't force you to follow a special diet, and a special diet isn't required to succeed. I would never perform a weight-loss surgery that forced you to follow a highly restricted diet against your will. What the surgery does is help you develop new habits, and you as the patient are the one who decides, over time, what those habits are.

Sadly, the concept of trying to force overweight people to follow highly restrictive eating patterns in order to lose weight is nothing new. However, as you're about to read, using surgery effectively will involve developing your own unique habits that work for you.

THE CLOAK OF DENIAL

The reluctance to admit that obesity stops you from doing things you'd really love to do is an interesting phenomenon that I've come to refer to as the Cloak of Denial. At first it seemed like an occasional phenomenon that I saw in my clinic, but over the years I came to realize that it's very prevalent, and in fact, it is more the rule than the exception. I see the Cloak of Denial when talking to someone who has desperately tried to lose weight, but then tells me, "I really don't think my weight is that big of a deal." Amazingly, I'm hearing this from people that come into my clinic seeking surgery in order to lose weight. The "it's really no big deal" rationalization is false, it simply doesn't fit their behavior.

The majority of American men and women spend time and money every year trying to lose weight. They buy pills that promise to help them lose weight in their sleep. They snap up the latest supplements to raise their metabolism or decrease their appetite. They purchase gizmos and gadgets that guarantee weight loss in a week. And they do these things over and over. So, why would they spend all this effort and money if being overweight was no big deal? Because it *is* a big deal, and they all know it. But sitting around all day and night, reminding yourself that you can't live your life the way you desperately want to, would be miserable. So, the Cloak of Denial becomes their coping mechanism.

"I didn't start becoming overweight until my early thirties, and my self-image never really adjusted. Every time I looked in the mirror, I expected to see the person I used to be, and no matter how often that expectation was dashed, I never stopped hoping to see that person looking back at me in the mirror, rather than the one I never really accepted or understood."

Sam B.
Screen Writer

You tell yourself that you're really OK, that it's no big deal, and it works to solve the problem, most of the time. The Cloak of Denial allows us to move on with life as best we can, in the shape we are in.

"Although the size of my clothes kept getting bigger, I must have had a magic mirror because I never saw myself as morbidly obese."

Carolyn O.
Real Estate Broker

And then, at some point, almost everyone allows reality in, and admits the truth. They stop the denial and accept the fact that *it's not OK*, that it *is* a big deal. That's when they look for a solution. If they find a promising possibility, they give it a try. Unfortunately, what often passes for promising solutions turns out to be only gimmicks or bad advice. So, they try these solutions but once they've lost the weight and gained it back again, The Cloak of Denial goes back on. To cope with yet another failure they tell themselves, once again, that it really *is OK* after all, that being fat is not a big deal.

"I've personally had many disappointing encounters with diets and appetite suppressants. I became friends with Jenny Craig, Nutrisystem, Weight Watchers, Curves, Slimfast, The

Grapefruit Diet, just to name a few. And, I became a tried and true friend of Dr. Atkins, more tried than true. Eventually I became the Queen of Denial. My mind knew that I absolutely didn't overeat, I could lose the weight. I could still fit in size 1X (tight), and surely I had a beautiful complexion. But, in reality, I couldn't even cut my own toenails, I had no self-esteem, I was depressed, and I had given up."

Sue E.

College Professor

The problem with this repeated cycle of sudden awareness, finding a solution, giving it a try, failing, going back into denial, then eventually finding another "solution" and repeating the cycle, has very little to do with you. **The problem is that the solutions aren't true solutions at all, and these false solutions simply become constant reminders of failure. The cycle beats you back into denial but without a reasonable solution, what else can you do?**

All my patients, every single one, have worn this Cloak of Denial at one time or another. It's normal, it could even be considered healthy...to a point. What's *not* healthy is to get up every day, look in the mirror, and call yourself fat, or to constantly remind yourself that there are many things you wish you could do if only your weight didn't keep you from doing them.

"It took me several years of contemplation to be ready to consider gastric bypass surgery. I had to accept the painful reality that I was morbidly obese."

Kim H.

Area Administrative Manager

Downplaying the significance is important for maintaining sanity, but at some point, you need to admit the facts to yourself and decide to either accept your current situation or take action to improve it. This book offers a different strategy from any of the "mainstream dieting strategies" you have tried. It offers a solution that can dramatically help you succeed. But in order to succeed I need you to be in touch with why you want to lose the weight. The *real* reason.

UNCOVERING THE *REAL REASON* TO LOSE WEIGHT

There are no commercials showing the joys of being obese. There are no movies or TV shows portraying how liberating it is to be so obese that it's hard to simply move around. All my patients tell me that when you're obese, it's just harder to move. It's hard to do simple things like climb stairs, get in and out of a car, and even to tie your shoes. I see the effort it takes most of my patients to simply get out of a chair and to get onto the clinic exam table. That's why there are no media messages showing us the pleasures of being obese and no commercials telling us how much fun it is to be fat. Because it isn't, and everyone knows it.

> "For many years, I was in denial about how big I actually was since I was still able to be somewhat active in the things I like to do. Although it was more difficult to get around."
>
> **Lisa B.**
> **Tax Resolution Analyst**

Commercials often show people we want to be like, doing things we want to do, making the friends we want to have, feeling the way we want to feel. They look active, fit, happy and free. Deep down inside, all of us want to be unrestricted in our ability to participate in life. Maybe not as a competitive athlete, maybe not as a swimsuit model, but on some level we want to be out there. We want to *do it*. We want to be active, to participate.

> "I gained weight again after getting married and starting a family. Then I was motivated to lose weight to become a firefighter. It was always easy for me to eat what I wanted and gain weight, then lose it when I needed to, going from one diet to another. By age 51, I was up to almost 300 pounds, had Type II diabetes and sleep apnea, and snored to the point my wife would sleep downstairs. I started to realize that I needed to take some permanent steps to get control of my health. I wanted to enjoy retirement, enjoy travel with my wife, and enjoy grandchildren. I knew if I didn't do something soon, I had a good chance of not fulfilling any of these dreams."
>
> **Edward G.**
> **Fire Chief, Retired**

The fact is, we all want to participate. For Edward, that meant being able to enjoy traveling with his wife and enjoy grandkids. For someone else, it means coaching a daughter's soccer team. Perhaps you dream of going hiking, stand-up paddle-boarding, or even competing in a local race.

The first step in getting there is to understand your true motivation, the real reason you want to lose weight. This requires

you to accept that there are things you want to do but can't because you're obese, and to acknowledge how important it really is not just to lose weight, but to be able to do what you truly want to do.

This is the real reason why you and almost all obese people want to lose weight. Your primary goal is not just to enjoy gazing upon your handsome reflection in the mirror, but to get out there and do something fun, to enjoy physical activity without restriction, to be able do rewarding and enjoyable activities with your family and friends. Fitness is a large part of the gift of life. It opens the door to the things we want to do and connects us with the people we want to do them with. It is an essential part of personal success. And in order to achieve future success, it's important to acknowledge that there are things you want to do but can't because of your excess weight.

This is hard for many people to admit, and that includes those who are constantly trying to lose weight. I've seen this over and over in my medical practice; it's a form of denial that most people are not aware of. They want to lose weight, they'd like to be fit, but they're reluctant to admit that being obese stops them from doing what they want to do.

INCREASING YOUR RANGE OF CAPABILITY

If your real goal in seeking weight-loss surgery is to be able to do things that you feel uncomfortable doing, or you simply can't do with all the excess fat, then the reason you want to lose weight is to "Increase your Range of Capability."

Look at the diagram below. You have a Range of Capability (your "Comfort Zone") that describes the range of things that you can do without struggling and suffering. Anything outside of this range takes you outside of your comfort zone. The problem is, this range is not enough to make you happy. As we discussed previously, you want to be able to do things that your weight restricts you from doing: play sports, join in outdoor activities, play with your children or grandchildren. In other words, your Range of Capability is too narrow.

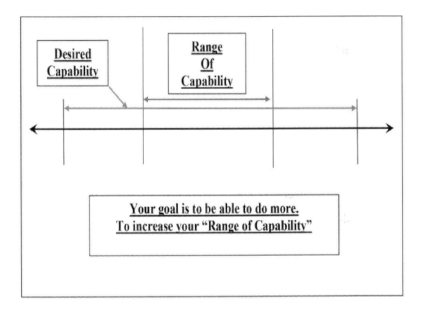

Losing weight will help, but will not automatically give you access to all those things that are currently outside your comfort zone. For most people, gaining a lot of weight didn't involve a lifestyle that kept your muscles toned, so your muscles aren't as strong as needed. Nor is your endurance as high as it needs to be in order to perform those things that are currently far outside your Range of Capability.

An example of this is something that comes up in my practice almost every week. A 30- or 40-something-year-old-woman tells me that if she could just lose the weight she would be able to be a "soccer mom" and play with her children and participate in their sports. I ask her how losing weight is going to result in increased strength and endurance. She then tells me, "I know, losing weight involves exercise, of course." Then I tell her that's not really true. Losing weight involves eating less, but becoming "fit" involves exercise. Then I ask her if what she's really looking for is increased fitness, and she smiles and says, "Yes, that's it."

This is good because the common ideas around weight loss are critical, they involve negativity; "I'm fat because I was 'bad' and I need to become 'good' so that I can lose weight." How miserable! I encourage my patients to try a better idea, to think of it this way: "I've decided to improve my fitness so that I can do really fun, cool things." Now that sounds a lot more positive!

So, the real goal, once again, is to improve your fitness, and this means exercise is part of the deal. Exercise, by definition, is outside of your comfort zone but, guess what, your entire goal is to do things that are currently outside of your comfort zone! So, you now have a choice; decide that you are sadly mistaken and you really don't want to improve your fitness, grab the remote control, pop a diet pill and hit the couch. Or, you can accept the fact that your true reason for wanting to lose weight is that there are things you're dying to do, things you believe are fun, and they will actually involve exercise to be able to do.

> "I'm 9 months out of my surgery and am concentrating on putting on more muscle. My diet is awesome! My weight has been holding steady at around 155-150 pounds. I eat tons of protein every day and even get to treat myself to some tasty treats since I train so hard. My results are unreal!!! I did a Brazilian Jiu Jitsu 'tourney.' Didn't win, but just competing was an accomplishment. I am also training for a paddling event to fight cancer in September."
>
> **Lou D.**
> **Vice President, D Enterprises**

THERE'S MORE TO IT THAN WEIGHT LOSS

All the people I know who are successful at staying fit do so because they want to take part in all the fun of life. They want to play, they want to participate, and they want to feel good while doing it. They don't want to break into a sweat climbing stairs or struggle getting in and out of their car. They want to fly on planes without a seat belt extender and shop for clothing at "normal" stores. There are a million reasons for fitness, and fit people work to stay that way because they want to live life without the restrictions imposed by a body that is holding them back.

> "It was the quality of life and the clothes. I mean let's be honest, okay? It's almost like you don't want to go out a lot because you feel like you don't look good, but when you feel

like you look good, you do want to go out and enjoy life. I love clothes, and I love fashion, but I couldn't enjoy it. I didn't enjoy getting dressed and going out."

Janice G.

Corporate Executive

Of course, we want to be medically healthy, too. We don't want to take medications for diabetes, hypertension or cholesterol. But let's face it, taking a couple of pills every day for high cholesterol or high blood pressure is relatively easy. It's not any harder than taking vitamins. And besides, even skinny people have diseases.

No, the main reason we worry about illness is that *it threatens our quality of life*. Once we begin worrying about diabetes causing blindness, or hypertension leading to a stroke, now *that* gets our attention. So, once again, we don't want physical limitations, we want to enjoy life.

"People ask me if I feel constrained now; if the surgery made me feel imprisoned in some way by the fact that I can never again binge the way I once did. Quite the opposite. I have been freed."

Sam B.

Screen Writer

It's critical for you to understand the true goal if you hope to be successful, whether you use surgery as an aid to achieve the fitness you seek, or some other method. I've discussed it, and provided numerous examples to underscore the truth. What you are really looking for is increased fitness and the better quality of life that comes with it. So rather than chasing weight loss in hopes that it will lead to the lifestyle you desire, I tell all my patients to pursue the active, fit lifestyle they hope for, and once they achieve that, their weight will be where they want it.

I tend to be a very visual person, and my patients often chide me for all of the drawings and diagrams I sketch out during consultations. I find that making diagrams of my concepts helps my patients visualize their goals and what they're trying to achieve. So, in keeping with that, I'm including my diagrams for the true goals of weight loss below.

Figure 1 (below) shows the FALSE GOAL of weight loss that focuses on achieving a certain weight that will suddenly give you the healthy, wonderful life you're waiting for.

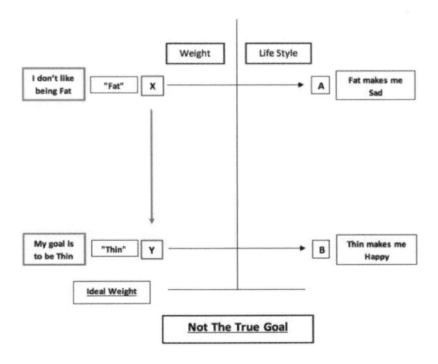

Figure 1: Weight Loss, the False Goal

Well, as I've explained, it doesn't happen that way, and most overweight people have dieted, lost weight, and have already found this out. If it worked that way, then everyone that lost weight on a diet would suddenly become happy and they'd go forward at their new "happy weight" forever.

Of course, after 20 years of listening to my patients tell me about one diet after another, this "happy forever" almost never happens, and we all know this.

Figure 2 shows the REAL GOAL of weight loss, which is to become fit by going after the life you really want.

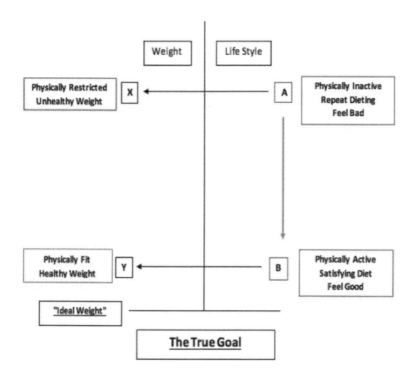

Figure 2: To Live an Active Life, this is the True Goal

By pursuing your active, healthy life, you will lose weight and you'll find that you are able to do those fun and exciting things that are your true goal after all. Then, once you find yourself "living the life," you can check your weight and you will find that the number on the scale makes you smile.

You want to live an active, fun life. To go from lifestyle A to lifestyle B. This is the real reason you're reading this book. If you pursue your true goal of increasing your range of capability instead of simply shedding pounds, you will find that you do get what you really want from weight loss, and you will have a reason to maintain your fitness, and your healthy weight, throughout your life. For my patients to permanently succeed with surgery, this concept is it. It's everything.

A LESSON I LEARNED FROM A PATIENT

Years ago, a retired Marine Corps drill sergeant came to my clinic and told me he wanted to have gastric bypass. Although he was clearly obese, he was also 68, and at that time most surgeons refused to perform bariatric surgery on patients over the age of 60. I asked him if he thought he might be too old to have the procedure. He looked down and quietly asked, "If I go under the knife, how long will it take me to recover from the surgery and then lose all this weight?" I told him the entire process would take about one year.

He looked me straight in the eyes and told me he had always lived an active life, until his weight gain made it impossible. Then he said, "I'm ninety pounds overweight and if I live five more years at this weight, I'll have five miserable years. But if I have surgery and lose this extra weight, even if I only have two more years to live at least I'll get one great year. I want that year."

That day, and many times since then, I learned a valuable lesson. People want to shed the bonds of obesity, and be able to participate in life so badly that they would be willing to trade a few years of a miserable life away in order to live a shorter but happier one. *Most people feel it's what they do with their life that matters, not how long it lasts.* It's a fact that's been repeatedly reinforced over my 20+ years as a weight-control physician. It's a reality that's at the heart of this book. While high blood pressure and diabetes will cause problems over time, inability to participate fully in life affects you next month, next week, and today. My Marine Corps patient taught me that **the main reason people hope to overcome obesity is because they want to participate in life.**

THE KEY TO SUCCESS

As a metabolic surgeon who has directed both medical and surgical weight-loss programs for decades, I have spent thousands of hours interviewing my successful patients to learn what they feel the keys to success really are.

What my patients have taught me is that obese people can achieve permanent weight loss by practicing the same simple principles that fit people follow. The difference is that people struggling with obesity are starting with a dual burden. Not only are they overweight, but they have to lose a lot of weight first just to be able to adopt the active lifestyle that would keep them fit. *Being obese prevents them from even starting the fitness program they need to follow in order to lose the weight and keep it off.* This is why they've chosen surgery, to finally lose enough weight and keep it off long enough so they can get on with the lifestyle that will give them permanent success.

The analogy I frequently tell my patients is this: Everyone needs to run a slow marathon throughout life in order to maintain a healthy weight, it's just that my patients must first climb over a mountain, before they are able to run the race. My job as a bariatric surgeon is to get them over the mountain. Running the race afterwards is still up to them.

Controlling your weight with the help of surgery can be straightforward, but it takes effort. If you are someone who has fought the battle of the bulge and lost it time and time again, it all starts by getting in touch with how you really want to live. By using some basic principles and the insight provided by my successful patients, you will be able to get your excess weight off, become happier and more fit, and maintain this success permanently.

WHY IT CAN WORK FOR YOU. OR NOT.

A comprehensive approach like mine is not rocket science. There is nothing magical or secret about it. The program I present in this book starts with surgery and then addresses multiple habits that lead to sustained fitness. They are the same habits that everyone who wants to live a long, healthy life must incorporate at some point, whether they are struggling with weight issues or not. The difference is, for many obese people, these lifestyle changes are simply out of reach. By undergoing surgery to help with the weight loss, a severely obese person is finally bringing these changes in lifestyle habits within reach.

But before you read any further, please be honest about your goal. If your goal is to ride a couch rather than to go bicycling, to sit on rides at the amusement park rather than to take a hike, or to watch travel shows on TV instead of exploring your world firsthand, then this book will be a waste of your time. This book is for people who want to lose weight in order to achieve something greater than being thin. This book is to help you become active, healthy and fit.

DECIDING ON SURGERY

By reading this book, you will see how surgery provided the initial leverage, and how successful people then took advantage of this leverage to achieve *and maintain* that healthy, happy and active lifestyle. I will show you how, after many years of dieting, they achieved the life they hoped for by following some simple, almost common sense, nutrition and exercise guidelines.

What is true for people who have maintained fitness throughout their life is also true for people who were, at one time, seriously overweight but have lost the excess pounds and kept them off. With or without surgery, the fact is that **both groups have discovered an active lifestyle they truly enjoy, and that keeps them physically fit.** It's not about dieting, nor is it just about exercise. It is both of those things, *and more.*

"Before surgery, I had heard people say the only regret they had was not doing the surgery sooner. I know what they are talking about and completely agree. With the gastric bypass and the skills that I have learned with The N.E.W. Program, I have the tools to keep the weight off for life. I will never be that woman who was missing out on her own life and watching from the sidelines. I am the woman living her life to the fullest!"

Michelle G.
Payroll Manager

WHY I DO IT

The short answer is, I do this because I have a solution that has proven effective. In over 20 years, I have helped more than 5,000 patients successfully reshape their lives.

After attending college for engineering and biology, I was accepted into the University of Minnesota School of Medicine. My formal education in weight-loss surgery started there (Minnesota was one of the first medical centers in the world to perform surgery for weight loss, in 1951), and I was first introduced to the science of obesity and metabolic disease in 1990. Professor Henry Buchwald, M.D., Ph.D., had just published a landmark study on intestinal bypass surgery to treat high cholesterol. I read it and realized right away how significant this was.

People around the world develop coronary artery disease and have heart attacks as a result of unhealthful levels of cholesterol. To prevent this, patients are prescribed expensive medications to control their genetic predisposition toward high cholesterol; these medications have numerous side effects and their success in preventing coronary disease is mediocre. Intestinal bypass surgery, according to Dr. Buchwald, proved far more effective. To me, it was enormously significant that an intestinal operation could have such a profoundly positive impact on a genetic disorder where pharmaceuticals were the only popular alternative.

Although I wanted to go into cardiac surgery where surgeons bypass clogged arteries, it seemed that controlling the underlying disease up front, rather than waiting until it had progressed, was more logical. I mentioned my fascination with this idea to several of the residents training in cardiology and surgery. Surprisingly, they all thought it was ridiculous that I would be interested in operations designed to help "fat" people. I had thought the significance of these operations was that they helped people with a metabolic problem—high cholesterol—but all that these other trainees seemed to be concerned with was the fact that the patient was "fat." I wondered, "What difference does that make?" but I realized that, to many doctors, the fact that the patient was obese was enough to ignore the science altogether. This was my first exposure to the deep bias against obesity in the world of medicine, and I've been bothered by it ever since.

I ran into this bias again during my surgical training at The University of Chicago. A brilliant professor, Dr. John Alverdy, was a skilled bariatric surgeon. The gastric bypass operations that he did were fairly simple, but the physiology involved and the management of these patients were complicated and interesting. Despite this, most of the surgical residents had little interest in this field. Nevertheless, I was intrigued.

A watershed event occurred later in my residency, when I met a ruggedly built six foot four fireman named "Frank." The man was about 240 pounds and clearly strong as an ox. I figured he must have been a heckuva lineman for his high school football team, and I thought to myself, "This is exactly the kind of guy I want climbing up a ladder to carry me out of a burning building!"

He was there for his annual check-up, and I immediately assumed that he must be there for some type of hernia repair. Surely this guy had never been sick in his life. When Dr. Alverdy stopped in the room to say hi, tears came to Frank's eyes and he bear-hugged him, nearly lifting him off the floor. After my professor and Frank had this reunion the man explained to me his story.

For most of his career, Frank had weighed about 230 pounds. He had always been a "big" guy, he said, but after about ten years with the fire department the stress seemed to catch up to him and he started having trouble with his weight. A promotion had landed him in a desk job with minimal exercise, and a bad diet had resulted in an expanding waistline and a host of medical problems.

The impact on his life was disastrous. Once he failed the routine physical required of all firefighters, he was put on disability. He tried "every diet known to man" but eventually got to 350 pounds. This made him depressed and he gained more weight. When his disability checks stopped, the financial stress resulted in his wife leaving him and taking away his two children. Divorced, alone, broke and over 400 pounds, he had considered suicide. But then he read something about surgery for weight loss and figured he'd give it one last try. His primary care doctor told him that he was "crazy" but he came to the clinic anyway, and later underwent a gastric bypass.

Now, three years later, he had lost close to 200 pounds and had been able to go to the gym (now that "everything doesn't hurt anymore"). He credited my professor with giving him his life back.

"I feel great!" Frank beamed. He explained how now that his extra weight was gone, he was fit and exercising, he was on good terms again with his children, was back to work as a fireman, and even had a girlfriend. This entire clinic visit took about fifteen minutes, and I walked out of the room amazed at what I had just seen.

With his story, Frank introduced me for the first time to the mental toll of becoming morbidly obese. He had been desperate to turn his life around, had tried multiple diets, and had been close to suicide. I remember feeling incredible empathy over what he endured as he lost the life he loved. I was dismayed by how he had been so alone in his struggle, with even his primary care doctor telling him that he was "crazy" to consider surgery. It was an epiphany for me, realizing that people like Frank are out there and they need help finding an answer.

One other incident in the weight-loss surgery clinic really impressed me. It was the case of a woman who had undergone gastric bypass surgery, but had regained the majority of her weight. She had undergone testing that showed everything about the surgery was working the way it was supposed to work, but the dietary survey had shown that she was now unemployed and sitting around at home all day eating potato chips and cookies. I saw her three times in the clinic and every time she had gained more weight, and every time she explained earnestly how none of it was her fault. She ate junk food all day because, as she put it, "It's the only thing that makes me happy."

I realized then that the difference between the highly successful bariatric patients and the profound failures was rarely the surgery itself, but was based mainly on what people did to make the surgery work long term. It seemed like what I was witnessing was a surgical field where specialized operations were being used to help people alter their lifestyle in healthy ways. Bariatric surgery was a mechanical modification that forced certain changes in eating patterns, *but was dependent upon the patient using these changes to alter their behavior* to be successful. Over the next several years of my training I saw similar stories, and learned as much as I could about bariatric surgery, or what I later termed Behavioral Modification Surgery.

The complexity of this field, the dramatic success when everything worked together, and the lack of understanding about what it really involved, all convinced me to devote my career to helping people manage their weight, not just through surgery or dieting, but through a comprehensive approach to weight management and wellness that would set patients up for permanent success. I didn't know it at the time, but this comprehensive approach was the foundation of The N.E.W. Program: Nutrition, Exercise and Wellness.

Now, 20 years later, I've treated everyone from celebrities and elite athletes to average Joes and Janes. I've studied the physiology, lifestyle patterns, psychology, and behavior patterns of obese people and healthy-weight people. And I have come to understand that people who are successful at maintaining a healthy weight often don't appreciate all they really do to maintain that weight. It is not just diet, but an entire lifestyle that leads to *fitness*.

My goal in writing this book is to educate you on weight loss and provide some guidelines for using weight-loss surgery effectively. Through insight from highly successful patients, you will see how people who have used surgery as effective leverage to get in shape have NOT had to adopt a lifestyle they hate in order to stay fit. Instead, they have found the lifestyle that they wanted all along, and which they genuinely *like,* now that they are able to practice it. **They've lost the weight by having the strength to**

pursue the life they longed for, first with surgery and then with a N.E.W. outlook, and have stayed fit because they like the lifestyle that keeps them there.

This is why I do what I do. It's more than just a surgical procedure; it involves working with hopeful and determined people that want to improve their lives. Bariatric surgery is a field that combines highly technical operations, science and lifestyle modification in order to achieve an amazing result.

WHY BELIEVE ME

I wrote this book backed by 20+ years of clinical observation and thousands of scientific studies reported in the medical literature. I've also included advice from real patients who have "been there," and then succeeded. During my years as a weight-control doctor, offering surgical and non-surgical weight loss counseling, I've interviewed thousands of weight-loss clients. I've observed their habits and studied the patterns that result in success or failure. As I observed weight-loss surgery patients become successful, I saw that the habits resulting in their success were the same habits followed by people who had maintained fitness their entire lives. It became clear that my job wasn't to come up with some strange and unique rule book that needed to be followed by "fat people" in order to help them lose weight; my job was simply to help weight-loss patients find their way to a fitness lifestyle. Nothing more.

TIME HAS PROVEN MY APPROACH

Early in my practice, in 1997, I began to perform bariatric surgery. With formal bariatric surgery training during my residency I turned out to be the only formally trained bariatric surgeon in the area. At that time, bariatric surgery was still considered a radical approach to weight loss and many doctors doubted my prospects for long-term success.

The first procedures I performed were all revisions or reversals of prior bariatric procedures that had resulted in one problem or another. What I noticed was that the patients being sent to me had undergone bariatric surgery without any real understanding of what the surgery entailed. None of the patients had been involved in a basic lifestyle education program prior to surgery in order to learn what their role was in making the surgery successful. It seemed that the surgeons that were in the field of bariatrics had gotten into the field by first doing the operation, and then patching together an after-surgery counseling and support group system. I decided that the entire field of weight loss, whether through surgery or not, was hugely dependent on the patient modifying his or her behavior. This, in my opinion, involved the patient understanding their role *prior to* surgery, and then choosing to participate in the system.

In order to provide this prior understanding, combined with post-operative support, I decided to first put together what I called a Nutrition, Exercise and Wellness program (The N.E.W. Program) and *then* to add on surgery, when patients chose surgery as their best option. Patients could choose either a surgical or a non-surgical path, and I had every patient set his or her own goals and identify the people in their lives that were capable of support. I made one additional stipulation that I felt necessary for success: **I insisted that each patient accept full responsibility for developing a combination of eating and exercise habits that would make the surgical approach successful.**

Were all my patients successful? No. No process can claim a 100% success rate. But this N.E.W. lifestyle approach, combined with surgery, was more successful than simply doing the surgical procedures alone, and far more successful than any diet-and-exercise program out there. Absolutely! And in the 20+ years since my first patient, I have personally developed a system that has resulted in success for thousands of overweight individuals.

TURNING THE CORNER

Denial is a powerful tool. But on the other hand, at some point, every one of my patients overcomes the Cloak of Denial I mentioned earlier, and admits, once and for all, that being obese is *not* how he or she wants to live for the rest of his or her life. This is when they get serious.

I'm not talking about your decision to renew that gym membership, or to buy another order of weight-loss food off the TV ad. I'm talking about a moment when you decide enough is enough, and you finally get *serious*. It is the moment when rationalization runs out and you no longer have a choice. This is the moment when you can't fake it anymore and you decide, no matter what it takes, your goal is *to succeed*.

> "Night after night, I would lay in bed and feel my heart fluttering and be afraid that I would have a heart attack or stroke, so I would promise myself that, 'tomorrow I will get serious.' I came to the realization that, by not taking care of myself, I could have serious medical complications and become a burden to my family. I was not willing to do that.

It took me several years of contemplation to be ready to consider gastric bypass surgery. I had to accept the painful reality that I was morbidly obese."

Kim H.
Area Administrative Manager

"Looking at family photos over the past 13 years you would have thought I did not exist. It was too painful to see myself in photos; I had to be the one with the camera in hand to avoid any shots of myself. My ongoing feelings of despair were repeatedly interrupted by periods of determination to get my life back. I committed to every diet imaginable, losing 100 pounds, 70 pounds, 90 pounds, only to gain it back again. Finally, after another forced diet plan failed, I decided that my last hope and chance to regain my life was to have a gastric bypass. I wanted to live a full and happy life with my children and at the rate I was going that was not going to happen. Instead, I had been literally killing myself."

Sandra L., R.N.
Director of Clinical Appeals

What is the breaking point? Everybody has a different one. I've listened to thousands of patients and though they say it in different ways, I've heard the same messages over and over again.

"I want to be able to get down on the floor and play with my grandkids."

"We go on a family vacation and I can't go on even a short hike because my knees hurt and I can't catch my breath."

"I used to love soccer. I haven't been able to play soccer for years, but now I can't even go to watch a game because I have so much trouble walking up the stadium stairs!"

"My doctor told me to consider jogging. Jogging! He's got to be kidding, I can't even reach down to tie on a pair of shoes!"

At some point the successful patient just decides to make the change to succeed. For many, this means coming to grips with reality. You want to be fit, you've tried hard, and you've failed. You aren't a loser, not at all, but the fact is, when it comes to weight and fitness, you have gambled and lost, sometimes repeatedly.

"Surgical weight loss was not an easy decision for me. Although obese for the majority of my life, I liked to believe that if I could only maintain a 'diet' I could control my weight. But after years of yo-yo dieting, hypertension, borderline diabetes, losing and re-gaining even more weight, I finally did my research and went to an information seminar at The N.E.W. Program."

Mary Ann E.
Assistant Deputy Commisioner

The reason you've failed at weight control is *not* that you can't do it, that you lack the willpower or are defective in some way. It's that you need a better strategy. My approach to bariatric surgery makes it the smart choice not simply because of the surgery, but also the pathway it opens up afterwards. Surgery opens up a window of time where a new lifestyle can be learned and can then become your habit. You *can* be successful without surgery, but for many people surgery provides just the leverage they need.

IT'S ALL UP TO YOU

The truth about successful permanent weight loss is that no matter what method you use, the long-term success *is completely up to you*. It's the same with bariatric surgery. It's not the easy way out and it doesn't guarantee success. Bariatric surgery is simply the most successful method for 1) losing a significant amount of excess weight and 2) using that weight loss to improve your life. This book gives you real insight into bariatric surgery and how to make it work for you. So, for those of you who want to live life without the restriction of excess weight, let's get going.

Section 3:

Preparing for Success

ESSENTIAL STEPS TO SUCCESS

After over 20 years of helping patients lose the weight they need to regain an active lifestyle, the steps to success are clear and predictable. These are the different stages in the process, and I describe each one in detail in the pages that follow.

(Section 3)
1. Commit mentally
2. Assemble your support system
3. Consider your insurance
4. Identify a surgeon
5. Attend your initial appointment
6. Pre-operative preparation and testing
7. Pre-surgery diet
8. Surgery
9. Post-operative recovery and healing

(Section 4)
10. Foods of choice
11. Dietary Rebuild
12. Exercise habits
13. Nutrition and Exercise

COMMIT MENTALLY
GETTING RID OF MISINFORMATION

News flash: Being thin isn't necessarily the best answer for you. Even if, medically speaking, you are at your healthiest when you're thin, it may not be wise to force yourself to achieve that "healthiest weight" if the lifestyle it takes to stay there makes you miserable. But, if you're not going to strive for your "ideal body weight," how do you decide what weight you really want to be? Simple: think in terms of your "*Best Weight*," the weight at which you are able to do what you want in life without having to persecute yourself through restrictive diet plans or extreme exercise to stay there. The point is that you should strive for a weight where you can live an active, healthy and happy life. Period.

> *"Your best weight is the weight at which you are able to do what you want in life without having to persecute yourself to stay there."* - Brian Quebbemann, M.D.

Diets are supposed to be short-term events. Athletes and body-builders go on a diet before a competition. Models diet in order to look a certain way for a photo shoot. None of these people go on a diet with the expectation of staying on that diet forever. It would be crazy to do so. It's simply not sustainable. You don't have a weight problem because you lack the willpower to stay on a perpetual diet, you have a weight problem because you haven't found an eating and exercise pattern that you enjoy that keeps you at your best weight.

When thinking long term, there are really only three main goals that people think about when trying to lose weight. See the diagram below.

The 3 Long-Term Goals of Weight Loss		
	Diet	Surgery
Appearance – The weight loss will help me look better	✓	✓
Health – The weight loss will help me be healthier	✓	✓
Quality of Life – The weight loss will help me enjoy life more		✓

Dieting succeeds with the first two of these goals. However, the most important long-term goal, and the main reason people come into my clinic looking for a permanent weight-loss solution, is the third goal, Quality of Life, and on this, dieting fails. The reason diets fail long term is because they are too restrictive, and people will simply not accept being permanently miserable in order to look better or to improve their health.

It's important at this point to define the difference between what I'm calling a *diet*, and what I refer to as your eating pattern, or *eating habits*. A diet is an all-out effort to lose weight. Diets generally don't take into account either the dieter's food preferences or his quality of life. Most often, a diet will define the goals for you, and then present a process for achieving those goals. *Eating habits*, on the other hand, are based on your personal goals and your food preferences, and are developed gradually over time.

You might be thinking, "Wait, you just told me that dieting is *not* the answer. How am I going to get to my best weight without dieting?" One answer is through weight-loss surgery. Surgery gives you a lot of *leverage* in your effort to achieve, and stay at, your best weight. This does not mean that weight-loss surgery is the "easy way out." The people that have failed to keep their weight off after surgery can attest to that. Most of those people assumed they could sit around, eat whatever they want, and still stay fit. They couldn't; they tried and it didn't work.

As a bariatric surgeon, I know that my surgical skills are important; I take surgery very seriously and I'm extremely good at what I do. But I also know that without my patients' full intent to succeed there is no chance of achieving long-term success. I need them to be in touch with why they are doing this, and we need a plan for achieving success. My patients and I are partners in this process, we are on the same team. I can do my part flawlessly, but without their effort we won't succeed.

The fact that my patients are ultimately responsible for their success is a good thing. When patients understand this, it empowers them. It reinforces their feeling of strength and self-determination to know that they have not "taken the easy way out," but instead have chosen a smart way out.

Now let's get on with how to make bariatric surgery work.

"It takes strength to show the world who you really are." - Brian Quebbemann, M.D.

YOU'RE NOT IN THIS ALONE (LIKE IT OR NOT)

It's your life, it's defined by your choices, you are the one who has to live with them. No one, whether family member or professional "expert," should be allowed to take ownership of what *you* do.

I once had a 50-something woman show up to a weight-loss seminar with her husband. After the presentation ended, I was answering questions from the audience and she explained that she had "tried everything" over the past 20 years: gym memberships, exercise trainers, vitamin shots, diet pills, commercial diet programs, and she had read multiple diet books. Now, morbidly obese, she wanted to consider surgery, but her husband was against it.

I looked at the man sitting beside her and asked him why he was against surgery. Her husband stood up, in the middle of the audience of about 30, and announced that his wife was "weak-willed" and she should just "commit herself" to being thin, rather than "pretending." He seemed angry. He was very skinny and a smoker—had already stepped out of the room twice to smoke cigarettes, and would hack and cough when he did. I could immediately see that her chances for success would be markedly undermined by this person.

Her tone, however, was clearly desperate, and I was touched by her sincerity. I asked her husband if he had tried to quit smoking. He sneered at me, "Of course." So, I asked why he hadn't been successful, and he said defiantly, "Because I like it!" Here he was, well on his way to an early death from emphysema, and "Because I like it" was his best excuse, and was also a way to say that his wife didn't truly want to lose weight. He then turned to his wife and told her, in the middle of the audience, that if she went forward with her plans to have weight-loss surgery he would divorce her, and then he stomped out.

The audience was aghast. One rather fit woman who was there with her obese husband turned and said "Honey, you don't need that man. You can come and live with me." The smoker's wife looked down, clearly beaten, and slowly walked out. I never saw her again.

Family has no monopoly on discouragement. Well-meaning friends, coworkers, and even physicians can prove to be unsupportive. One example occurred while I was giving "grand rounds" (an educational seminar for doctors at the request of a hospital) about ten years ago. The topic was diabetes and obesity, and how to treat both diseases using surgery.

I had invited along two successful patients, both former diabetics, who had used surgery to lose their excess weight and to resolve their diabetes. One patient was a bank president, the other a grade-school teacher. Both were about four years out from surgery, and after my presentation, they shared their inspiring success stories with the audience of almost a hundred physicians. Both patients explained their multiple efforts at weight loss, their difficulties treating their diabetes, and their eventual decision to have surgery. They also discussed how their lives had finally turned around after gastric bypass, with loss of most of their excess weight and the resolution of their diabetes.

When they were done, I asked the audience if anyone had questions. Among the crowd were three physicians in their mid-sixties who had been whispering and chuckling during most of my seminar. The middle one raised his hand and asked, "Why would you do surgery when these people really just need to see a psychiatrist?" (This is a true story!)

I had just given an hour-long seminar on the causes of obesity and diabetes, and being crazy was not a cause. I had discussed alternative methods for treatment, reviewed statistics on the efficacy of surgery and had two happy, *successful* patients (both thriving professionals) for whom surgery provided a successful solution, explain their stories. Then, after all that, I got this insulting question, from an experienced physician, no less.

The lesson from these two episodes is that a misunderstanding of the issues of being overweight, and the negative bias that comes with it, know no boundaries. This lack of support comes from people who are *unwilling or incapable of opening their minds to a surgical solution.* It can be from your committed life partner or even from a medical professional. And this negative bias can represent an almost insurmountable obstacle to finding and committing to a solution. The good news is, with the increased awareness about the hazards of excess weight (and the abysmal success with non-surgical weight loss), a growing number of people are sympathetic to your struggle.

When it comes to unsupportive people, whether they are your friends, family or your physician, you need to somehow move beyond them in order to succeed. Find a few people—and you only need a few—that truly, deep down inside, support you without limit or reservation. These people will be open-minded on various methods of weight loss, including surgery. They simply want you to succeed. And, once they've heard your story, or maybe they already know it, they will support you in whatever method you choose to pursue.

This is your support team. You need one.

"People, even those who care for you, will expect you to fail. Help like this you don't need. This is *your* experience; share your efforts and goals only with people who are materially invested (in your success) and you should know that this list is remarkably short."

Gwen S.

Corporate Partner

ASSEMBLE YOUR SUPPORT SYSTEM

You might be thinking "I'm going to do this on my own" and maybe you can, and maybe you will. But make no mistake, there are a lot of messages you receive every day that affect how you think about yourself, how you set your goals, and what you think you need to do to achieve those goals. Some of these messages come from commercials, marketing companies or social media, others come from people you know and trust. The problem is that no matter where these messages come from, they can affect how you think. And when it comes to weight loss, everyone thinks they have "the answer."

When you identify a team, you identify those people whose messages you *trust* and whom you can rely on for *positivity and consistency* when you are going through the weight-loss surgery process. It's also important to understand the role of each person on the team. Everyone on your team is not an expert in obesity or in permanent weight loss. Do not include people that *think* they are an expert unless they are truly an acknowledged expert in the treatment of severe obesity and have a track record of success. For example, your personal trainer is an expert in physical training but is generally not an expert in how to succeed after bariatric surgery. Even a supportive spouse may not be your best support unless you both understand that the role he or she plays is not that of an expert.

I've had obese men come in with their overweight wives who want surgery, and the husband tells me that his wife is there because "she needs to lose some weight." I look at him, with *his* seventy extra pounds, and I ask him what he's going to do about his weight. Generally, the wife jumps in at this point to "protect" hubby. "He doesn't really have to lose weight, he's always been a 'big guy,'" she says. I ask her how long they've been married and she smiles and tells me, "Twenty-eight years. We were high school sweethearts." Then, I ask hubster how much he weighed when they got married, and he proudly responds, "I was 190 pounds back then. Running back on the football team." At this point I mention that he's now pushing 260 (I'm an obesity expert, remember, I can guess your weight) and I ask him, "So, the additional seventy pounds that you have gained since you got married must be all muscle. Have you been weight lifting quite a lot?" I then get a slightly guilty chuckle out of hubby and he admits that he could do with a bit of weight loss as well.

I then steer the couple toward the concept that maybe a partnership, improving their fitness level together, would be a good thing. Most of the time they clearly like the idea. Part of the reason it comes across as a positive idea is because the goal is *fitness*, not "weight loss."

When it comes to advice on all matters relating to bariatric surgery, the main experts on your team must be your surgeon and his/her team of professionals. Think of them as your professional support team. Of course, your primary-care physician needs to be part of this team as well. An unsupportive physician will not work.

Bottom line is that nobody is automatically on your team. Not your family, not your friends, not your physician. You need a *completely* supportive team, and you should be careful who you choose to be on it. All people on your team must see your success as the ultimate reward and must be willing to support you and your efforts, *even if they don't completely understand.*

Finally, in the end, you need to believe in yourself in order to make permanent weight loss work. This is vital; the most important person on your team is you.

DO AWAY WITH UNSUPPORTIVE PEOPLE

Just as assembling your support team is important, so is watching out for Unsupportive People. They might not be who you think they are. They might fool you.

The unsupportive people you should avoid are the people who, when they hear that you've decided to have weight-loss surgery, start the sabotage. For some reason, they do not want to see you succeed, at least not this way. In my clinical practice I've seen examples of this many times. A classic one is the husband that takes you on an all-you-can-eat cruise a month before your scheduled surgery. Or the spouse that shows up after surgery with a two-pound box of chocolates. This is a problem that happens more often than you might think, and when I see this I intervene on behalf of my patient immediately. However, we don't always win. In the end, the only person who can remove the unsupportive saboteurs in your weight loss quest is you.

"Lack of support and outright antagonism comes from friends or even your physician. My friends all felt that surgery was dangerous and that it was 'the easy way out,' and my physician was completely opposed to it. This is why I didn't tell any of them that I scheduled the Lap Band surgery until the day before I did it. I decided to take responsibility for myself; to date, none of them can believe the results. My physician admitted he was going to have to re-examine his position."

Joe K.
Regional Sales Manager

SUPPORT VS. EXPERTISE

There is a big distinction between helpful support and expertise. The treatment of obesity and the science of weight loss are very complex. Unless a person has formal training and experience in the science and practice of weight control, they are NOT experts in the treatment of obesity.

One common mistake is to rely closely on a friend who has succeeded with weight-loss surgery, and who believes that this makes her or him an expert. It does not; it only makes her a successful *patient*. You wouldn't think that a person that has survived a heart attack is now an expert on coronary artery disease, or a person that has overcome cancer is suddenly an expert in cancer treatment.

People who have succeeded after bariatric surgery are very aware of their experience as a weight-loss surgery *patient*, and that experience may be something that can help you. If your friend's goal is to support you, and not to play the expert, then they could be a helpful part of your team. However, if someone without the required training considers themselves to be expert on obesity, weight loss or bariatric surgery, then you're best off not having them on your team.

A Dr. Q Story

Weight loss has always been an intriguing field for me, in part because there are so many so-called "experts." It's funny how almost everyone thinks they know how you should lose your extra weight. I was in San Francisco at a bariatric surgery conference years ago, and to get back to my hotel I jumped on one of the trolleys. As I was riding along, searching for my stop, the hugely obese trolley operator, who must have seen some papers I was carrying, suddenly announced to me and anyone within earshot that the answer for weight loss was to cut out all red meat and carbs. "That's the trick!" he said. And he smiled after he said it, with full knowledge that he—at roughly double his ideal body weight—had just provided the Holy Grail of weight loss to his passengers.

This reminds me of a quote by Bernard Baruch, Wall Street broker and presidential advisor: "Beware of barbers, beauticians, waiters—of anyone—bringing gifts of 'inside' information or 'tips.'" And his admonition applies to all the self-appointed experts out there: "Don't speculate unless you can make it a full-time job."

Professionals can lack expertise, too. I've given hundreds of presentations and seminars to patients, families, community groups, nurses, hospital administrators, and physicians over the years. The most stubborn group has always been physicians. One question I've been asked by physicians, on many occasions, is "Why should I take any responsibility for the fact that some patients choose to be fat?" I love this question, precisely because it's so uninformed. My simple response to this question has been to ask the doctor the following question in return: "Have you ever heard of a 12-year-old child who, when asked what he wanted to be like when he grew up, responded, 'I'd like to be morbidly obese'?" In fact, there are probably few things that a child would fear more than being an outcast due to his or her weight, and the expression on the face of the physician that asks this question usually betrays this awareness. And so, I follow my first question by asking, "Then why would you pretend that your patients *have chosen* to be obese any more than others *have chosen* to have diabetes?"

It is important to identify your team, identify the roles of the people on your team, and to use this awareness to help eliminate unsupportive people from your inner circle of fitness. Once you have done this, you will be ready to proceed forward in the weight-loss surgery process.

THE WEIGHT-LOSS SURGERY PROCESS: FIRST STEPS

Now that you've decided to proceed with surgery and you've identified your team, there are basic steps in the process from the time you decide to make an initial appointment, through to your recovery after surgery. You've decided to see a bariatric surgeon in consultation, but your first step forward in getting bariatric surgery is *not* calling to make your appointment. The first step is to do a little research concerning your options.

CONSIDER YOUR INSURANCE

If you plan to use medical insurance to cover your surgery, you will be restricted to only those surgeons who have signed contracts accepting whatever your insurance company is willing to pay. If you are insured by an HMO, then that HMO will have an even more limited number of surgeons either working for them, or contracted under their plan. This limits your options, but this does not mean that your options are bad. There are qualified bariatric surgeons working under contract with private insurance plans, PPOs, HMOs and with government insurance. They might not be the surgeon that you feel is "the best of the best," but many of them will be trained in bariatric surgery and will be safe and skilled.

Nevertheless, there are certain things you need to ask before making that call to set up your first appointment.

IDENTIFY YOUR SURGEON

• <u>Does your surgeon specialize in bariatric surgery?</u> Is bariatric surgery something that he/she does frequently, or is bariatric surgery just a small part of his/her overall practice? The greater percentage of a surgeon's practice that is devoted to bariatric surgery, the more often that particular surgeon is focusing on how to perform it correctly. My practice is essentially 100% bariatrics, but this is rare, and I know several excellent surgeons that perform bariatric surgery frequently, but not exclusively. The point is, some degree of specialization is important.

• <u>Is your surgeon a *Fellow of the American College of Surgeons* and a *Fellow of the American Society for Metabolic and Bariatric Surgery*?</u> Being a Fellow in these societies requires both board certification and ongoing professional education.

• <u>Is the hospital or center where the surgery will be performed a designated Center of Excellence (COE)?</u> There are two organizations that designate COEs. The first organization to designate Centers of Excellence was the Surgical Review Corporation (SRC) and currently the largest organization designating Centers of Excellence is the American College of Surgeons (ACS). Both organizations are good. If the center is not designated as a COE, it might still be OK, but having the formal designation as a Center of Excellence is a big plus.

- <u>Does your surgeon offer long-term support?</u> They can provide the support themselves (some individual surgeons provide excellent follow-up) or they might have a support team that handles long-term support (some teams are excellent). Either way, long-term support is important.

- <u>How many bariatric surgeries has your surgeon performed as primary surgeon?</u> This means that the surgeon actually did the surgery; being an assistant in surgery doesn't count. The bare minimum I recommend is 200 cases as primary surgeon. You are best off with a surgeon who has performed over 1,000 bariatric surgeries as primary surgeon.

- <u>Has your surgeon performed a significant number of Gastric Bypasses and Gastric Sleeves during the past year?</u> The Gastric Bypass and Gastric Sleeve are the two most common bariatric procedures in the world, with the highest benefit-to-risk ratio. If your surgeon does not perform both of these procedures regularly, then you should ask for a good explanation as to why.

If you were able to answer "Yes" to all of these questions, that's a good start. This doesn't mean that the program is automatically excellent, but it does mean the program has put in considerable effort to provide a quality service.

One fact that is important to keep in mind: Any surgeon can claim to be an expert, claim to have performed "thousands" of surgeries, and even tell you that they are "world-renowned." Unfortunately, surgeons report their own statistics, training and expertise, but the information they report might not be accurate.

Examples of warning signs:

• A surgeon who claims to be "world-renowned." If you are world-renowned, you don't have to tell people this.

• A surgeon who claims to be a bariatric expert, but has limited or no experience in one of the main procedures, Gastric Bypass or Gastric Sleeve.

• A clinic where just one procedure, the Gastric Sleeve, the Gastric Bypass, The Lap-Band™, or the Duodenal Switch is miraculously the "best procedure" for everyone. This is usually because the surgeon is not competent in the other procedures.

• A clinic that is reluctant to refer patients for procedures outside their area of familiarity. I sometimes think that a procedure that I do not perform (Duodenal Switch, for example) is the best procedure for the patient. In these circumstances, I refer that patient to a surgeon that performs the Duodenal Switch.

Look for solid experience and a sense of honesty and forthright behavior in your surgeon. The vast majority of surgeons will have your safety and success as their top priorities. Good results, extensive experience, formal training and specialization are all good. In the end, however, you will need to trust your instincts.

ATTEND YOUR INITIAL APPOINTMENT

After you've done your research, you need to call and make an appointment. If you are a member of an HMO, you have limited options in specialists. If you have a choice based on a private insurance plan, or if you are willing to pay cash for your surgery, you will have many more options.

All experienced bariatric centers will be able to verify your insurance benefits and counsel you on your options. It can be difficult for you to get accurate information from your insurance company, and sometimes difficult to find out what requirements your insurance company has put in place before they will pay for your surgery. Experienced bariatric centers can answer these questions for you.

> A Dr. Q note:
>
> Always ask the center if the bariatric surgical procedure itself, not just the pre-operative testing, is covered by your insurance, AND ask if your surgery will be covered by your insurance *at their center*. I've heard of centers that have a bait-and-switch game going on. One example of this is to tell you that "you are covered" and then they perform numerous tests, for which they get paid, only to tell you at the end of the testing that they are unable to take your insurance for the actual surgery you want. Another example is when the center is not contracted with your insurance company but does not inform you of this up-front; they string you along, and then at the very last minute, claim that they were "unable to get your insurance approved" and tell you you'll have to pay cash. Sadly, there are dishonest physicians and institutions out there, so just beware of these situations before you fall into a trap.

Most insurance plans cover bariatric surgery! In fact, it is rare these days to have a plan that excludes bariatric surgery as a covered benefit. Just remember, your insurance is *your* insurance, and you are obligated to accept the requirements that your insurance company has put in place.If you are unhappy with the regulations imposed by your insurance company, you might be able to successfully challenge them. There are legal experts who might be able to help; one such law firm for Obesity Advocacy can be found at ObesityLaw.com.

Current Standard Insurance Requirements for Bariatric Surgery:

1. Morbid obesity:
   a. BMI (Body Mass Index) of 40, or higher
   b. BMI between 35 and 40, with specific weight-induced medical problems

2. A three- to six-month documented attempt to lose weight, with monthly dietary consultations, at some time during the past two years

3. Clearance for bariatric surgery by a clinical psychology professional

If you choose to go through your insurance, it will often take effort and diligence on your part. If you can afford to pay cash for your surgery, then you will have complete choice on where to go, who to trust as your surgeon, and when to have your surgery. This is truly a life-changing event, and having some control over who does your surgery might be well worth it.

PRE-OPERATIVE PREPARATION AND TESTING

Now that you've called for your appointment and you understand your insurance coverage, the clinic will likely send you educational materials. *Be sure to read the materials.* This is your chance at success; take charge of it, this is not a game.

At your first appointment, you will probably meet your surgeon. If you do *not* meet the surgeon at your first appointment, this is a warning flag. This means that the surgeon doesn't want to be bothered until the very last minute, so they don't have to waste their time on you.

Personally, I won't go to a surgeon that does this. In my surgical training I was impressed with the fact that the surgeon knows more about the surgery than anyone else, and so, as a patient, I want to hear everything he or she has to say. But this is up to you. Some programs have information seminars to go to first, and this is not a bad thing. However, early in the process you should expect to meet the expert.

Every center has its own pre-surgery process. The process my clinic follows is below in a flow diagram. Individual experiences may vary based on your medical conditions, your BMI and other factors, but the overall process will generally flow as shown below. This entire process can be completed in less than one month or may take several months, depending on payment method and patient preparation.

PRE-SURGERY PROCESS:

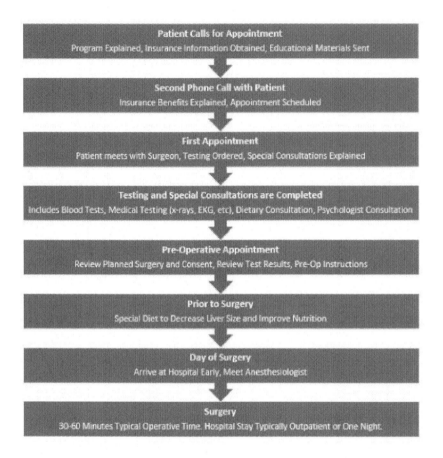

Patient Calls for Appointment
Program Explained, Insurance Information Obtained, Educational Materials Sent

Second Phone Call with Patient
Insurance Benefits Explained, Appointment Scheduled

First Appointment
Patient meets with Surgeon, Testing Ordered, Special Consultations Explained

Testing and Special Consultations are Completed
Includes Blood Tests, Medical Testing (x-rays, EKG, etc), Dietary Consultation, Psychologist Consultation

Pre-Operative Appointment
Review Planned Surgery and Consent, Review Test Results, Pre-Op Instructions

Prior to Surgery
Special Diet to Decrease Liver Size and Improve Nutrition

Day of Surgery
Arrive at Hospital Early, Meet Anesthesiologist

Surgery
30-60 Minutes Typical Operative Time. Hospital Stay Typically Outpatient or One Night.

PRE-SURGERY DIET

This pre-surgery diet is vital to your safety at the time of surgery. All patients must follow this diet in order to undergo surgery. The pre-surgery diet:

- Decreases the size of your liver, improving safety during surgery
- Helps to stabilize blood sugar

A Dr. Q story:

When I first started doing laparoscopic bariatric surgery, it was apparent that the markedly enlarged liver of most obese patients was going to be a problem. Early in medical school we are taught that the liver stores fat and a fat-like substance called glycogen. We are also taught that most of the glycogen and a lot of the fat will be metabolized quickly (over several days) if a patient is subject to starvation. I also noted that many patients would have a "last supper" the day or two prior to surgery, falsely thinking that they were never going to be able to enjoy eating again. The "last supper" syndrome, as I called it, would result in rapid accumulation of fat, making the liver massively swollen at the time of surgery. I realized that this practice of gorging on food prior to surgery was making the surgery much more difficult and risky, since the liver covers the stomach and had to be moved (if possible) out of the way in order to perform the procedure.

To me, this was like a goose being force-fed in order to accumulate fat in its liver in order to make foie gras. It seemed reasonable to put patients on a diet immediately before surgery in order to decrease the size of the liver. Since starving patients for several days prior to surgery would be a bad idea due to possible electrolyte and sugar imbalance, I decided to have patients follow a very low-calorie diet (called a VLCD) for two weeks prior to surgery. This worked quite well and my problems with an oversized liver abruptly ceased to exist. I also found that patients with diabetes came in with much healthier blood sugar levels, making the administration of anesthesia safer.

In 2003, I was attending a bariatric surgery meeting in Bethesda, Maryland, when the chairman of the meeting mentioned that the most common cause for converting a laparoscopic (minimally invasive) procedure into an open (traditional big incision) type of surgery was the extreme size of the liver in bariatric patients. He then gave an example where he had to convert from a laparoscopic procedure to an open procedure, and even then, found that the liver was too big to complete the gastric bypass. He had then abandoned the planned surgery and told the patient that their liver was too big to undergo gastric bypass safely.

I was aghast. Here we were, the "big people surgeons," and we told some patients that they were too big to undergo surgery? I got up and went to the microphone and explained my two-week VLCD protocol, and said that I had been using it for two years with excellent success. I made the mistake of jokingly calling it my "anti-foie gras diet" and many of the surgeons laughed, and nobody seemed to pay much attention. After my comment, however, two academic surgeons (one from Davis, California and one from Australia) came up and asked me for my protocol.

Despite the early doubts that I encountered, and a few surgeons suggesting that I was simply using the protocol to sell nutritional products (I did not sell products in my clinic at that time), many surgeons now use a similar protocol, and hepatomegaly (enlarged liver) has all but ceased to be a problem with laparoscopic bariatric surgery.

The basic protocol that I use for my pre-operative Very Low-Calorie Diet is described below. This diet is designed only for a very short timeframe, and is not meant to be continued for more than several weeks. I typically use this diet as a two-week pre-operative diet, but occasionally extend the diet to three or four weeks for certain super obese patients who have massive livers prior to surgery. The goal of this diet is simple; it is used to improve visibility and safety during surgery. If a patient refuses to do this diet, or shows up on the day of surgery and admits that they have not followed the diet, I cancel their procedure and tell them to find a new surgeon. Patient accountability is critical for the success of bariatric surgery, and this applies to the entire process including the process prior to surgery.

Diet Protocol

1. Never go more than two hours (during the day) without eating or drinking

2. **High-protein, low-calorie shakes.** Drink two shakes per day (women) or three shakes per day (men), 30 grams protein/shake

   - We recommend Premier Protein (purchase at Costco or Sam's Club) as a quality commercial brand, or Bariatric Advantage brand High Protein Meal Replacement (ordered online)

3. **Calorie-Free fluids.** Drink at least 64 oz. of calorie-free fluids per day

   - Examples: water, Crystal Light, vitamin water, unsweetened tea

4. Vegetables. Eat only the non-starchy vegetables listed below (no other vegetables allowed)

- We recommend that you eat at least three servings of these vegetables (each serving should be at least four ounces, or ½ cup) every day. You may eat up to six servings. You can eat them raw or cooked. Adding spices is OK.

- Bell Peppers
- Lettuce
- Celery
- Cucumber
- Radishes
- Carrots

- Spinach
- Cauliflower
- Broccoli
- Onions
- Kale
- Brussel Sprouts

5. **Additional Protein**. Eat <u>one serving</u> of additional protein daily. Choose one of the three options below.
- Tuna, five ounces (about one can)
- Chicken Breast, five ounces
- Beef or Turkey Jerky, three ounces

6. **Nutritional supplements**. Use high-quality supplements, usually those made specifically for bariatric surgery patients.
- "B Complex," one dose/day; multiple B vitamins including B-12 and B-1 (Thiamine)
- Vitamin D, 5,000 IU daily
- Multivitamin, 1 dose/day
- Iron
- Calcium

The day before surgery you should take in clear, sugar-free liquids only. This can include broth, Sugar-Free Jell-O, water, tea, light coffee without creamer, Diet Sprite, and other clear, calorie-free beverages. This will help to empty out your stomach, making the surgery safer.

SURGERY

On the day of surgery, you will arrive several hours early in order to fill out paperwork and get processed through to the surgical preparation area, called "Pre-op." In the pre-op area, the nurses will run some minor tests (check your vital signs, etc.), start an I.V. and sometimes give medications. You will meet the surgeon and anesthesiologist who will answer any of your last-minute questions.

The surgery itself generally does not take long. Highly skilled surgeons will take anywhere from thirty to ninety minutes to complete your actual surgical procedure. Speed is not the main goal, but completing the surgery correctly and safely is. The best surgeons do not brag about how fast they do surgery, but they also do not waste time. The team of operating room personnel is critical in making sure that everything the surgeon needs is available.

The anesthesiologist is responsible for comfortably putting you to sleep, keeping you stable during the procedure, and waking you up again after surgery. The anesthesia process typically takes approximately 10-15 minutes before surgery and 10-15 minutes after surgery. Once surgery is completed you will be taken to the recovery room. The anesthesiologist typically oversees the nursing care in the recovery room (called a PACU, Post-Anesthesia Care Unit) after surgery. You will typically remain in the recovery room for one to two hours after surgery; here the nurses will monitor your blood pressure, heart rate and breathing. The nurses will also be in charge of administering pain medication. It is normal to have some pain after surgery and the nurses should have experience in what is a normal pain level, as well as when to administer pain medications. Once the nurses in the PACU feel you have recovered adequately, you will either be discharged to home (if you are planned for *outpatient* surgery) or transferred to the hospital ward (*inpatient* surgery).

Recovery after laparoscopic (minimally invasive) surgery typically involves mild to moderate post-operative pain for one to three days, after which you should require only liquid Tylenol for your discomfort. Every patient has a different "pain threshold" and recovers from surgery in a slightly unique way, but in general you will be completely off all pain medications after one week. Open surgery, where a single large incision is used rather than several tiny incisions and cameras, requires much longer for recovery, but is no longer a common way to perform bariatric surgery.

> "My expectation after waking from surgery was I'd be in a lot of pain. In reality, any pain was negligible, akin to having done a lot of sit-ups several days in the past. I was quite surprised by the almost absence of pain."
>
> **Doug S.**
> **Business Owner**

Immediately after surgery you will be taking in liquids only; this allows you to get in adequate hydration and nutrition while your new anatomy heals. Within a few weeks you will be instructed to eat soft foods as a transition between liquids and regular food.

Once your surgery is completely healed you will be able to eat regular foods, but you will have to chew your food well and eat slowly.

After minimally invasive surgery, the healing of your incisions (the skin and the muscle beneath) is fairly rapid. I tell my patients that they can typically be back to "normal" activity within 10-14 days after surgery. At that point, they can move around and lift things without hurting themselves or tearing open the incisions.

The above brief description of your surgery day, and your immediate post-operative recovery, is meant only as a general overview. Every surgeon has his or her own process and protocols, and your surgeon will provide you with specific instructions to follow based on what they believe is best for their patients.

It is important to remember that your surgery, and the several weeks it takes you to recover after surgery, should *not* be thought of as a period of weight loss. The main goal during the surgery process is to set up your anatomy in a way that enables you to lose most of your excess body weight *over the next six to 24 months*, and then keep that weight off for years, hopefully the rest of your life. The immediate post-operative focus of you and your surgeon should be to do everything necessary to help you recover in a way that ensures proper healing. Again, weight loss is *not* your primary focus during recovery; the primary focus is healing. Once your surgery is healed, you can then turn your attention back to weight loss and improved fitness.

POST-OPERATIVE RECOVERY AND HEALING

Once you have completed surgery, you will be in the recovery and healing phase of the process. Recovery from the surgery varies slightly between the different procedures, but there is a general length of time needed to allow the surgery sites to heal, both external incisions and internal changes to your stomach anatomy. The total length of recovery and healing time is roughly thirty days, or about one month.

The diet progression varies from surgeon to surgeon, and there are no hard and fast rules on which protocol is the best. I have my own protocols developed out of my understanding of how the gastrointestinal tract (stomach and intestine) heals, and based on years of feedback from my patients on what is comfortable one, two and four weeks after surgery.

Remember, the goal immediately after the surgery is not "weight loss," but rather the promotion of healthy nutrition while allowing time for the surgery to heal.

The stomach is much smaller following surgery, and there is some edema, or swelling, of the stomach lining which will temporarily distort the stomach anatomy. Taking in solid foods during this time could increase the risk of getting food stuck and rupturing the stomach, possibly resulting in an emergency situation and even the need for re-operation. This swelling should be reduced substantially after two weeks. In order to allow your new stomach anatomy to heal without undue stress, I ask all patients to follow a progressive diet that begins with liquids only, changing to soft foods after about two weeks and then changing to regular food after four weeks.

Excellent nutrition can be maintained within those first two weeks after surgery using high-protein shakes, high-nutrition meal replacements, pureed soups, homemade smoothies and other supplements. In addition, many other liquids are fine to drink while on the two-week post-operative liquid diet.

My post-operative dietary protocol immediately after surgery (during healing) is really quite simple:

- Take in *liquids only* during the first two weeks after surgery. These liquids can be anything. In fact, I use the phrase "If it pours, it's yours." I tell people to *avoid solids of any kind during these two weeks.*

- Drink protein shakes daily (two shakes/day for women, three shakes/day for men, using shakes with 30 grams protein/shake).

- Drink additional unsweetened liquids. Examples include nonfat or 1% milk, unsweetened soymilk, G2 Gatorade™, soup that has been pureed in a blender (drink only soups with a broth base, not a cream base) and other sugar-free, non-carbonated beverages.

- Highly recommended to drink one quart of "Dr. Q's World-Famous Smoothie" each morning.

- Do not eat any solids (meat, whole fruits or vegetables) or soft foods (such as scrambled eggs, yogurt, oatmeal or cottage cheese, pudding or soup with whole chunks of chicken) during this Phase-One, liquid diet.

- Your minimum daily *protein* goal is 80 g/day (women) or 100 g/day (men). Protein is needed for safe healing.

- Examples of healthy liquids include tomato soup, low-calorie Gatorade, vegetable beef soup *that has been pureed in a blender*, fruit smoothies with added protein that have been made a bit thin and watery.

The problem with solid foods is that your stomach has narrow sections where thick foods may pass through slowly and be uncomfortable. Whole chunks of solid food could get stuck, resulting in vomiting or a more serious complication.

I've seen programs that promote formulas to calculate "exact" protein needs, and use other complex protocols after surgery. I am educated enough on the physiology involved to understand it, and I can tell you that keeping it simple, and focusing on what's truly important is your best plan of action. Once the initial two weeks (14 days) of healing have been completed, patients can usually begin to eat soft foods. This enables patients to continue healing while learning how thoroughly food needs to be chewed.

By four weeks after surgery, the sutures and staples used to change your anatomy are no longer needed and your stomach will have healed adequately to withstand normal intestinal stress. At this point, you should start eating "normal food." Normal food means exactly that: normal, typical types of food that people eat every day. This does not mean that you should eat unhealthful food, far from it, but it means that at this point the choice is yours, and you won't cause injury to your new anatomy *as long as you chew well and eat slowly.*

In my program, my goal is to return patients to normal, everyday food as soon as reasonably possible. The surgery was done to help you modify your eating and to learn a new healthier eating pattern while losing all that excess body fat. So, getting safely back to eating regular food as soon as possible is the goal.

A short, true story:
In 2002, I performed a laparoscopic gastric bypass on a very intelligent, morbidly obese attorney. The procedure went well, she was discharged to home with the Phase One Diet

Instructions, and my clinic called her on Friday, four days after surgery, to see how she was doing. She was doing great and the dietitian reinforced to her the 14-day liquid diet instructions and activity recommendations.

That weekend I took a drive up to Santa Barbara for a much-needed one-night-away at a nice hotel, where I expected to get some rest and some family time. At 9:00 PM on Saturday, after dinner and settling in for the evening, I received a call from the emergency room at my hospital—the attorney from Monday was in the ER with severe abdominal pain and a massive intra-abdominal infection (called an acute abdomen with septic shock).

I jumped out of bed immediately, threw on my blue jeans and T-shirt and drove 95 mph back to Orange County, getting a speeding ticket along the way. I got to the hospital, and found my patient in a lot of pain and developing a severe abdominal infection. I told her that we had to go back to surgery immediately to fix whatever was wrong internally. After giving her strong pain medication, I asked her what had happened. She admitted to me that she had been "doing so well" after surgery that she felt she could eat anything she wanted, and so she cooked a panful of grits (she was from the South) and sat down to devour them. After eating about six big bites she realized that the grits were "stuck" in her stomach. She developed severe retching and vomiting but the grits remained stuck. Apparently, she retched for two hours and then suddenly "felt something rip" and immediately developed abdominal pain. She called 911, and by the time she got to the ER the pain was severe.

I took her back to surgery, and found the stomach ripped open along one inch where sutures had been placed. I also found that every surface of every anatomical structure in her upper abdomen had been essentially sprayed with partially-digested grits. I repaired the ripped portion of the stomach, left the grits where they were (impossible to get them out, and they would be absorbed anyway) and she recovered quickly.

My "family weekend break" was ruined, but the patient re-covered without incident. Needless to say, she followed all of my protocols to the letter thereafter.

Copies of my pre-operative and post-op dietary protocols, "Dr. Q's World-Famous Fruit Smoothie," my Basic Nutritional Guidelines (BNGs, for use when back on a regular diet), and some other pro-tocols are included at the end of this book.

SECTION 4:

ACHIEVING YOUR BEST WEIGHT

THE THREE PHASES OF SUCCESSFUL PERMANENT WEIGHT LOSS

Successful *permanent* weight loss, where you come away with the power to maintain a happy weight without the constant oversight of a weight-loss professional, involves three main phases.

They are:

- Phase 1 – Weight Loss
- Phase 2 – Transition
- Phase 3 – Weight Control

The diagram below provides a schematic depiction of the phases involved in permanent weight loss after bariatric surgery, and also a depiction of the pathway followed by yo-yo dieting. For success with permanent weight control, each of the three phases is important, and each has certain nutritional principles to consider. Understanding this will help ensure long-term success.

In this diagram, I plot out three lines:

1. A theoretical line showing your Best Weight
2. A pathway showing the typical weight pattern followed by the Struggling (Yo-Yo) Dieter
3. An ideal line for long-term weight control after bariatric surgery

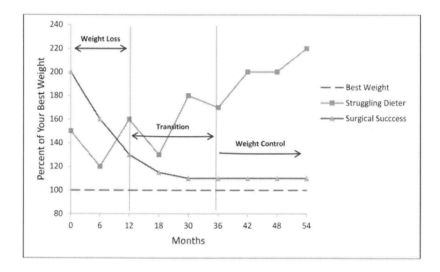

The first phase is the **Weight Loss** phase. This is the phase that everyone thinks about when thinking of a diet. Unfortunately, it's the *only* part of the weight-control process that most people think about, and this causes a huge problem. Weight loss, especially dramatic weight loss, requires you to be in a very calorie-restricted state, relative to your activity, or calorie expenditure. In other words, you need to take in (eat and drink) *far fewer calories than you burn*. A weight-loss period like this is not meant to be continued forever. Taking in fewer calories than you're burning is hard to sustain for long, and can be unhealthy. Of course, taking in fewer calories than you're expending will eventually make you sick, weak and mentally exhausted. So, the principles followed during the Weight Loss phase should be only adhered to during that portion of the permanent weight-loss process. In order to achieve dramatic weight loss, or to continue weight loss over a long period of time, it is best to work with a weight-loss professional.

The second phase, the **Transition Phase**, is possibly the most critical phase in the entire process, and sadly it's the phase nobody seems to think about. It is during this phase that patients rebuild their dietary habits. This is where you practice modifying your diet to one where you are eating food you still like, *but you are also following an eating pattern that doesn't cause your weight to climb*. After surgery, your appetite will be reduced during this phase, making it much easier to find sustainable eating habits; it's one of the main ways your surgical procedure helps you keep the weight off permanently, so use it to your advantage! When you've dieted before, you've probably struggled with overwhelming hunger, and you've been focused on weight loss at all costs, making it almost impossible to find a new sustainable eating pattern.

With bariatric surgery it's completely different. During the period of time your appetite is reduced, you *need* to eat highly nutritious foods in order to maintain your health. As a result, you are practicing eating healthful, nutritious foods *right away* after your weight-loss surgery...and you're doing so without being plagued by hunger. You lose weight rapidly and, if done right, you will move through the Weight Loss and Transition Phases seamlessly, *without* doing the Personal Persecution Program thing. And when your hunger goes back up a bit, you have lost much of your excess weight and have developed more enjoyable and nutritious eating habits along the way.

The third phase is **Weight Control**, often called "maintenance," and it's talked a lot about in diet books. The problem with this phase is that most dieters, and diets, get this phase wrong; they carry over the restrictive mentality from the Weight Loss phase and try to continue with this forever, and it's not sustainable. Many diets don't actually recommend continuing with a calorie deficit, or in other words consuming fewer calories than you are burning off, but they do persist with a "restriction" mentality. Some of the terms used a lot are "portion control," "foods to avoid," "count calories," and other "don't go there" rules. This is the "persecution" mentality that people just can't seem to live with.

> "I was always made to think that what I needed in order to lose the weight was more willpower. I don't call it willpower, it was 'won't power' because it always came down to the things I should not eat, not drink, it was 'don't eat more than this amount,' 'don't eat more than this many calories,' on and on. All the diets did was force me to constantly think about what I couldn't have, shouldn't do, until I got tired of it and just ate everything that I was told I should not want."
>
> **Denis S.**
> **General Contractor**

The key to the Transition Phase is that you find a lifestyle, eating pattern and an exercise pattern that you actually enjoy. This phase is where the real power of weight-loss surgery becomes apparent because you will continue to lose weight, without experiencing overwhelming hunger, and you will have an opportunity to choose an eating pattern that will help you maintain a *permanently* healthy weight. The most important part of the weight-loss process begins once your healing phase has completed, and it' important that you make the most of it.

One admonition that I tell all of my weight-loss surgery patients: if you spend your time after surgery trying to get back to the eating pattern that got you here, you will succeed, and you will eventually end up at that same weight again. The goal is to find a new eating pattern, not to return to your old one. My unique Dietary Rebuild™ method makes this process easy.

The Struggling Dieter

Before explaining the guidelines for maximizing your success with surgery, I want to describe what *not* to do by explaining the graph of the Struggling Dieter (seen in red).

The Struggling Dieter focuses entirely on weight loss. His goal is simply to "get the weight off" and he's often willing to try just about anything in order to succeed. This usually means following a very restrictive diet in order to cut down on calories. The need to cut calories in order to lose weight is very real, but a problem arises when you think *this is all there is to it*. As the dieter goes on he finds out two things: one is that staying on a highly restricted diet gets ever more miserable as time goes on, and the second is that he has nowhere else to go, there is no plan other than to remain on this diet for life. This mentality is why I refer to many diets as Personal Persecution Programs (a "Triple-P"). The Triple-P is not compatible with a happy life, and everyone eventually abandons this and returns to their previous eating pattern, and the weight comes right back on. To make this pattern even worse, this process is progressive, and the peak weight typically gets higher and higher with each subsequent attempt.

Unfortunately, the pattern of the struggling dieter is very real for too many people. I mention it briefly here so you can remember it as a pattern that you need to avoid in order to achieve long-term success.

<u>Surgical Success</u>

A successful surgical solution (the green graph line) to weight loss describes a consistent path of predictable weight loss. Losing weight rapidly in the months following surgery (while you are consuming much smaller portions), your weight loss tapers off in the Transition Phase (as you rebuild your diet habits), and flattens out (once you reach your best weight) in the Weight Control Phase. (Weight often rebounds up *slightly* from its lowest point, before stabilizing; this is common and nothing to be concerned with.) It is a proven path, and one which my successful patients can follow indefinitely.

FOODS OF CHOICE

"In our evaluations before surgery, we are told over and over again that this surgery isn't magic. But it is. The transformation is completely magical; it's just that the magic requires a lot of hard work after its initial 'overnight' effects."

Samuel B.
Screenwriter

Here you are. You've gone and done it. You decided it was time to quit messing around with diets, you had the surgery, and you recovered. It's been five weeks since your surgery and your surgeon told you that you're "doing great." You were on a liquid diet for two weeks to allow the surgery to heal, you transitioned through a period of soft foods and you are now starting to eat regular food. Not only that, your surgeon said you can start regular activity. Your surgery has healed.

"Wow!" you think, "That was fast!" and you are now starting to wonder, "Now what the heck do I do?!" The confusion sets in, caused by repeated efforts at dieting, different dietary books with completely different rules, multiple different diet formulas from high-protein liquid diets to the meat-and-bacon Keto routine to the vegan diets… It all suddenly comes back, and the chaos starts to set in, and you wonder "What the heck do I do now!?" You think, *this is a weight-loss program so…* What do I eat?

- How do I eat?
- When do I eat?
- How do I drink?
- What about coffee?
- What about wine?
- What about snacks?
- Where is the rule book, how do I do this?

You're starting to get worried, and your biggest worry is *"What if I eat the wrong things and the surgery doesn't work!?"* Not only that, your bariatric surgical program instructed you to start regular exercise.

- What do they mean by that?
- How often is regular?
- How hard can I work out?
- Is walking the dog enough of a workout?
- Do I need to join a gym?
- Why do I have to exercise? I thought I was going to lose weight because of the surgery.

All of these questions, and many more, have been asked hundreds of times every year in my clinic. I get asked these questions after surgery even though I discuss all of this prior to surgery, and provide written instructions.

The fact is, before surgery there is simply an "information overload" issue that all patients face. The surgery, and everything surrounding it, is something that your surgeon and the bariatric program team deals with every day. We are professionals and this is what we specialize in, so understanding the science and the process is easier for us. But for you, the patient, this entire program is a completely new experience, and the fact is there's A LOT involved.

"Take responsibility for your outcome. Over-communicate with your doctor when things feel wobbly, you are worried, don't feel well, get discouraged, want your money back. The onus is yours to diligently report your progress and engage your doctor."

Gwen S.
Corporate Partner

All the questions above are legitimate questions, but the best way to answer most of these questions, and start you on your road to success, is to simply explain the guidelines and instructions I provide for my patients. By understanding these guidelines, you'll be able to make good decisions and good choices *on your own*, and you'll be able to proceed down the road to success.

RULES?

After years of dieting, most of my patients don't trust themselves to follow a healthy eating pattern without someone giving them specific instructions. For most of my patients, every time they've committed themselves to losing weight, there was a set of diet rules to follow.

These questions are the questions of a chronic dieter, what I call the "Recovering Dietolic." They are the result of years of brainwashing by a diet industry that sells incomplete or false information and achieves pathetic results. This brainwashing, and the resulting addiction to diet rules, is a problem in my clinic.

The one main problem is the underlying belief that "fat people need to become better at following diet rules if they are ever to become skinny people." It's such a prevalent problem that I've considered hosting Support Groups for Recovering Dietolics.

Interestingly, if I ask my obese patients why they got to be so overweight, most of them will be at a loss for an answer. When they do finally answer, they tell me that they just have a lack of willpower, that they "know" the rules, and they say, "If I could just stick with the rules I would be thin." Well, as I said before, there are really no rules that work for everyone all the time. Most of the fit people I know follow healthy patterns, but very few of them follow strict *rules* for eating.

The good news is that you don't have to follow a strict set of rules to make weight-loss surgery work. This is a good thing.

"The goal of surgery is not to change your anatomy so that you are forced to avoid eating. And surgery is not a means of forcing patients to follow a strict diet.

There is nothing magical about surgery that suddenly changes bad diet advice into good advice." - **Brian Quebbemann, M.D.**

Being told to buy certain size plates, to cut your food into tiny pieces, to eat X ounces of protein and Y grams of carbs, to put your fork down between each bite, to chew thirty times, and other rules are, in my opinion, absolutely ridiculous. So, you're supposed to ask waiters to bring tea saucers for you to eat from, you chop your T-bone steak into a hundred pieces on your plate, you weigh out the amount of fish allowed. Really?! You've got to be kidding! Nobody healthy follows rules like that and I'm not going to pretend that my patients should either. My goal is to get patients back on track to being normal, healthy people, empowered to make *their own* choices for maintaining a healthy weight, not to turn them into unhappy social freaks that follow strict rules to limit their food choices and calorie intake.

Examples of absolutely goofy rules that I've heard, and never understood:
- You should eat this many calories.
- Don't eat more than this volume of food.
- Never use a straw.
- Avoid all carbonated beverages.

These and other goofy rules float around the weight-loss surgery world. If you ask for the science behind these rules, there isn't any. NONE WHATSOEVER! Unfortunately, these rules confuse people by focusing them on meaningless things and serve mainly to make the weight-loss program gurus feel that they have provided "good diet advice."

You will NOT get these rules here.

I also won't provide you with a bunch of recipes; I'm a surgeon, not a chef (although I'm a damn good cook!). You can find some excellent cookbooks filled with healthful recipes written by award-winning chefs. My advice: Buy one.

My goal is to get you to your Best Weight, and *give you the insight you need in order to choose your own healthy lifestyle*. I want you to decide what to eat and to take control over *your own* weight and fitness. You can't do this by blindly following a set of specific diet rules. The core of your success depends on *you* determining what works *for you*. You don't need to base your eating on what worked for someone else. With a little understanding and the right choices, you can develop your own healthy pattern of eating.

WHAT IF...

If the state or country where you live ceased to exist, and you suddenly were forced to move to another place, where the only food available was quite different than the food you now eat, most likely, you would be able to find a new eating pattern and develop new habits, and still be satisfied with your eating. So, **don't believe for a second that the way you used to eat, the eating pattern that put on all your extra fat, is the only way of eating that you can**

possibly enjoy. Thinking that way is naïve and ridiculous. Worse, it will doom you to failure. If you believe that your current eating pattern is the only one you can enjoy, then forget about successful, permanent weight loss altogether. I mention this, one last time, so that we are on the same page going forward. Your goal is to find an eating pattern *that you enjoy* that is *different* than what you've done in the past.

NUTRITION: EAT WELL

I want *you* to decide what to eat, and to take control over *your own* weight and fitness. You can't do this by blindly following a set of specific diet rules. The core of your success depends on *you* determining what works *for you*.

So, how do the common operations used in bariatric surgery help patients change their eating habits? ("Common operations" include the Gastric Bypass, the Gastric Sleeve, and the Gastric Band. I am not referring to the Bilio-Pancreatic Diversion nor the Duodenal Switch, which are not common operations.) The answer lies in the fact that these operations have a profound effect on your appetite, your sense of hunger, and even your sense of smell. The end result is a major impact on how you think about food—my patients have been telling me this for years, and I believe them. These effects are not the same in everyone, but the important point is that the effects of bariatric surgery can be used to modify your eating habits.

"The most astounding change in myself is that ALL MY CRAVINGS FOR SWEETS ARE GONE! I AM NEVER

HUNGRY, now I eat for nutrition and survival, and I make much better choices with the food I eat! I don't feel deprived, or like I'm on a diet! Basically, I can pretty much eat what I want, with one or two restrictions, but I feel full with very little amounts of food now."

Cheryl B.

Preschool Teacher

The effects of bariatric surgery that I have found to be the most useful to my patients are these:

1. You will have Less Appetite
2. You will Feel Full with Smaller Meals
3. You will have to Chew Well
4. You will have to Eat Slowly

LESS APPETITE: "THE HONEYMOON PERIOD"

Loss of appetite is a remarkable thing. It's not that you will get an aversion to food, but you will simply experience a period where you have no appetite. This effect can occur with the Lap-Band System, but it's much more consistent with the gastric bypass and the gastric sleeve. This is commonly referred to as the Honeymoon Period, and it generally lasts about six months after either the gastric bypass or the gastric sleeve. It can be as brief as only two to three months, or I've seen it last for several years.

We aren't completely clear on why patients have less appetite. Scientists debate the impact of removing a part of the stomach versus bypassing it, and they discuss the impact of hormones such as ghrelin and others. The bottom line: the precise mechanism for the sudden lack of appetite after surgery is unknown. Nevertheless, it occurs in the majority of surgical patients and is a very useful effect.

This period of markedly decreased appetite makes the bariatric surgery process completely different than dieting. You don't have to try to avoid eating, as you do during a diet. Since your appetite is reduced, you need to be more mindful of the need to eat, and you need to eat highly nutritious foods in order to maintain your health. As a result, you are practicing eating healthful, nutritious foods right away after your weight-loss surgery. You lose weight rapidly, and go through the Weight Loss Phase and the Transition Phase without being plagued by hunger. And when your hunger eventually increases a bit, you've lost much of your excess weight and have developed new eating habits along the way. How cool is that!? No wonder so many people are so successful long term after having weight-loss surgery!

It is critical that you focus on getting adequate nutrition during this period of decreased appetite. I go over this multiple times with every patient that goes through my bariatric surgery program. You must focus on taking in enough nutrition and drinking enough fluids to maintain your health. You need adequate nutrition in order to maintain your lean body mass (muscles, bones, internal organs) while you are eating so few calories and losing weight rapidly. Since you feel much less appetite, you should keep track of how much food you are taking in, in general, and be sure to drink enough calorie-free beverages to stay well hydrated. In addition, all patients are instructed to take daily vitamin and mineral supplements. My program personally recommends one brand of highest-quality nutritional supplementation because there is such a wide variation in commercial supplements. Many cheaper supplements are a waste of money, and the high-quality supplements are excellent. (All of my patients must agree to follow the nutritional supplementation guidelines, otherwise I refuse to perform their surgery.)

During this honeymoon period of decreased appetite, now is the time to experiment with eating different foods and different flavors. My Basic Nutritional Guidelines are provided in order to help with this transitional process, but the bottom line is that, without a lot of hunger, you are able to practice eating for good nutrition and good flavor. This process can be summarized by the term "practice." You are practicing a new eating pattern that is based on the quality of food and not the quantity. If you use this period effectively, you will come out the other end with new eating habits that will enable you to maintain a healthy weight for the rest of your life.

> "I did not need an audience for every food choice or setback and certainly did not want unsolicited advice—'You are so beautiful at any weight, who needs it?' 'You should try serious dieting one more time,' 'You know you could die on the table'—and I also knew my good success would be self-evident in time. And it's much more difficult to argue with success."
>
> **Gwen S.**
> **Corporate Partner**

SATIETY, FEELING MORE SATISFIED WHILE EATING LESS

An important physiological key to why the anatomic change is important, is that the upper portion of your stomach, called the "cardia," sends signals to your brain telling you that you are *satiated* (no longer hungry, or "full") when food passes through. After any of the three types of surgery discussed in this book (Bypass, Sleeve, Band), the food you eat feels like it remains in your stomach for a longer period of time, resulting in more signals telling you to stop eating. *This means that you get more satisfaction from a smaller amount of food.*

For most people, this is a dream come true. Now, instead of your mind telling you how you "should" eat, and your body telling you that you're still famished, your mind and body work together. Remember that every weight-loss coach out there preaches that an important factor in controlling weight is to be more thoughtful when eating. Often called "mindful eating," it's a fundamental principle with successful weight control. After one of these surgical procedures, you *won't* need to continuously tell yourself to stop eating, you will literally be signaled by your stomach that you are no longer hungry. What you *will* need to do is to pay attention to your body and make sure that what you eat has some nutritional value to it. Often, it takes a bit of getting used to, but all of my highly successful patients use the feeling of early fullness and satisfaction to practice eating differently, and they succeed.

CHEWING WELL

People like to chew. Chewing is something that makes us feel good. Apparently, the act of chewing (and other repetitive muscle activity) seems to give off endorphins, which are short-acting hormones that go straight to your brain and make you feel good.

Think about it; we sometimes chew gum, and when the flavor is gone, we don't automatically spit out the gum. When you see someone walking along chewing on a piece of gum, ask yourself, are they chewing that gum because they want to exercise their jaw muscles in hopes of burning off a few extra calories? The answer is they chew gum because they *like* to, it's calming and satisfying. So, it stands to reason that a surgery that encourages you to develop a habit of chewing more will result in you feeling more satisfied with less food.

Before surgery, people can choke down food that's been barely chewed and the stomach will grind it up and process it before passing it on to our intestine for absorption. Although few of us eat that way, almost everyone has experienced a moment when they realize they've swallowed something before it was chewed properly, and it feels "stuck." It's very uncomfortable. We don't do this very often because we learn how uncomfortable it is the first time, and we pace ourselves thereafter. This is a natural mechanism, we don't have to think about it, and chewing our food properly is already a habit.

After any of the three common bariatric procedures this learning mechanism still works, only it works a lot better. Your food must be chewed very well in order to comfortably pass through the narrow part of stomach that has been created. If you don't chew well you will get a feeling similar to not having chewed your food at all. Because you are chewing more with each bite, you will be tasting your food more and you will be more mindful of the flavor and quality of the food you eat. The best thing to do with this situation is to eat good-tasting, flavorful food, and learn to enjoy eating for the quality of what you eat *rather than the quantity*.

This may not be a dramatic change, since most people already get uncomfortable if they don't chew properly. But surgery does shift the situation significantly so that people learn to chew every bite a lot better.

EATING MORE SLOWLY

After surgery food will generally feel as if it passes through your stomach more slowly, so you will have a tendency to eat much more slowly. You won't need to quickly gobble down large quantities of food. Although the reasons differ based on the procedure you've had (Gastric Band, Gastric Sleeve, Gastric Bypass), food will feel like it passes through the upper portion of your stomach *slowly*. If you try to eat quickly, by not listening to the signals to slow down that your stomach is sending, you will get to a point where your food "gets stuck." If you still persist in trying to force food down, you will have to regurgitate, or vomit the food back up. Nobody likes to do this, and if this happens everyone learns not to repeat it.

In several studies, people who ate more slowly tended to be more satisfied with smaller meals. This has always been an interesting fact for me because, in my medical specialty, I'm frequently dealing with patients who eat quickly. When I ask them why they eat so fast, they sometimes look at me as if I'm a bit naïve and tell me, "Because I like to eat, Doc." Then I ask them why they eat too much and they tell me, "Because I'm never satisfied."

Now, think about this. They eat quickly in an attempt to satisfy themselves, but they are still never satisfied. Hmmm? Maybe the method they're using to satisfy themselves is not working. What if they tried a different approach: they approached eating by finding really tasty food, that required a lot of chewing, and then they ate those foods slowly, chewed it well and savored the flavor? Most experts will agree that, if people ate this way, they would tend to be satisfied with less food and we'd have less obesity.

PUTTING IT ALL TOGETHER

So, after your weight-loss surgery you will have a system that results in less appetite, you feel satisfied with smaller meals, and your body will remind you to chew well and eat more slowly. As a kid from the seventies I want to say, "Holy Cow, Batman!" I mean, this is great stuff! Think about it, your body is now working to support you in being a more mindful eater and still enjoying what you eat. This has been, after all, the goal of every diet you've ever been on. Now, all you have to do is practice, and soon these effects will work without you always having to think about it.

> "Your love affair with food is over. It will never caress you, soothe you, amuse or entertain you in the way it has before. But also true, you will never hate or fear food again either. Food becomes pleasant sustenance; it's fuel. If you are not prepared to break up with food, turn around—'surgery' is not for you. Personally, I knew I had many years of loving food behind me and I was truly ready to move on. I wanted something new to love."
>
> **Gwen S.**
> **Corporate Partner**

For people who eat more than they need to, or eat faster than they need to, and who have tried unsuccessfully to modify their eating for years, surgery is a game-changer. Subconscious signals to your brain are now curbing your appetite, telling you to slow down as you eat, and telling you that you're full after eating a very small portion of food. You now have much more power to modify your eating habits into ones that won't cause weight gain. You will need to focus on food that provides healthful nutrition, and since you're only eating a small amount of food, you can afford to be picky and only eat foods that truly taste great. So, here you are, focusing on eating nutritious foods that taste great, and losing weight rapidly, without having to spend the entire time hungry.

THE THREE-S RULE

Many diets promote some type of pattern of intermittent starvation. This requires you to spend your life in the Hungry Zone, or worse. Diets that counsel you to practice portion control as a specific goal, count all your calories, or strictly avoid certain types of foods, will often leave you feeling deprived, perpetually hungry or "starved." You try hard to stay on the strict regimen but you get hit with numerous negative side effects such as constant hunger pangs, headaches, feelings of weakness or tiredness, and cravings. When you just can't take it any longer you "cheat," which means that you fail.

This "cheating" or "failure" is simply you giving in to the signals that your body is giving you to eat. With this feeling of being a failure many people will simply decide to "eat whatever I want" since "I've failed anyway." Many people will say, "If I'm going to cheat, I might as well cheat in a way that makes me happy." This feeling of being deprived results in an overwhelming drive to eat, and many people start to believe that this abnormally high hunger drive is "normal" for them.

The result is that you eat whatever gives you a feeling of immediate satisfaction; you eat fast and blow right past the feeling of being satisfied, and you don't stop until you get to stuffed. You may have failed but at least you're not starved, in fact you're stuffed. Since the solution involved overeating and getting stuffed, you begin to think of being stuffed as the goal. Over time, you get used to this stuffed feeling and this feeling of being stuffed becomes your new eating goal. Then, if you try to lose weight again, you try to use willpower to force yourself to stay feeling starved, to live in the uncomfortable zone.

This back-and-forth process is miserable, but it's something I've seen frequently in my clinic. Patients come in who are living their entire life outside of the comfort zone and in the misery zones of feeling either starved or stuffed.

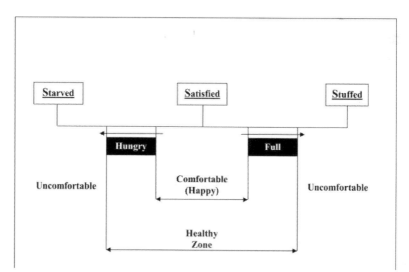

Dr. Q's Three-S Rule

This diagram demonstrates the 3-S Rule, a concept that has been useful for me in diagramming for patients what *not* to do, and helping them understand their goal.

After surgery, you will have a new opportunity to teach yourself about eating. My recommendation is to stay within the "Comfortable" zone *at all times*. Never allow yourself to get too hungry and don't eat until you are overly full. Once you have healed from surgery, and you are back on normal food, think of this diagram when you are deciding on when to eat, and how much to eat, during the day.

Feeling stuffed is not fun. I've discussed it with hundreds of patients; they are uncomfortable when they eat too much, but it's a habit that's hard to break. It's similar to a hangover after a night of drinking—you think you're having fun while you're over-indulging, but afterward you pay the price. A statement I've heard many times is "Doc, I can't wolf my food down anymore." And my response is, "Great!" I've asked many patients, "So, when you're very full, or stuffed, do you feel comfortable enough to go on a walk?" and they all say "No." One patient actually responded, "Doctor Q, that's what the remote control is for, so I don't have to move after dinner."

Feeling satisfied with less food, in combination with the need to chew well and eat more slowly, is a very powerful tool that helps people modify their eating habits permanently. It's normal to enjoy eating, and remember that the goal after surgery is to find that *new eating pattern* that you enjoy, but that will *not* pack on the pounds.

DIETARY REBUILD

A structured tool to use in discovering a new eating pattern that you enjoy is something I call the Dietary Rebuild. This is an optional process for many patients, in that there are other ways to achieve the goal of replacing your old normal with a new eating pattern after surgery. For others, my Dietary Rebuild provides a structured approach for redefining your eating habits and achieving your goal.

"DIETARY REBUILD"

The Dietary Rebuild is my answer to a chronic problem that patients have always struggled with. This problem involved them trying to walk through to the development of new, healthful, non-weight-gaining eating habits after their initial rapid weight loss and once they are back on regular food. Essentially every patient will lose weight rapidly after surgery, especially while they are on a post-operative liquid diet with high-protein supplements. During the initial healing period after surgery, the weight loss is rapid. After about four to six weeks, patients are typically able to transition to regular food.

Once back on regular food, my clinic has always coached patients on what foods to focus on and why. The recommendations include high-nutrition-value foods that are satisfying. These are mostly unprocessed as well as minimally processed foods, high-fiber foods, high water content foods, and natural whole foods.

The problem I've always encountered is that as soon as my patients return to "normal" foods, they are hampered by their prior understanding of what normal is. For people who struggled with obesity, the food they normally ate is the food that brought them to the point of needing bariatric surgery in the first place. So, the patient is again stuck with the situation where dietitians, doctors, nutritionists and others are telling them which foods to avoid, which foods to minimize, and which foods are "bad." For patients that have undergone bariatric surgery after going through multiple previous diet programs, this sounds an awful lot like the dieting advice that they were stuck with in their multiple previous failed attempts at weight loss.

It became obvious that my patients were struggling with a history of their "normal" diet (eating pattern) prior to surgery serving as their baseline. And, they were using the surgery to *avoid* diets! So, once again, despite all the benefits of surgery, we were in a different form of a Personal Persecution Program, possibly easier to implement due to the benefits of surgery, but with a lot of rules, negative messages about food, and an effort at restricting intake nonetheless.

To solve this problem, I implemented a program that would *reset* my patients' baseline, and I call it a <u>Dietary Rebuild</u>.

Your eating pattern before surgery bears no relation to your situation after surgery; you had more appetite before, you could eat much faster, and didn't feel full with small meals. So, looking back at your eating prior to surgery, and calling that your "normal," is now ridiculous. Using your previous normal as a baseline, and working backwards to modify that previous eating pattern in order to succeed with surgery, is pointless. The problem is, however, what will be your new normal? Every patient will have a different normal, so starting with a prescribed eating pattern that fits every patient isn't possible. The solution is a Dietary Rebuild that helps you identify your new normal; a normal that will serve as your baseline for the future, that won't result in weight gain, and which you can modify *as you see fit*.

Dietary Rebuild is a structured process that is not designed for weight loss, and is not a diet (I use it in my non-surgical program as well). It is something I use to coach my patients to an eating pattern that is fundamentally healthful and satisfying, but is also personalized for each of them. By using this process, you throw out all the eating habits you had before surgery, since they have no relationship to the present. I start you with a basic nutritional platform, and then rebuild your baseline eating habits back into something you like and that you can succeed with long term. This is the essence of the "Dietary Rebuild Program." I start you with a broad, but very well-defined, eating pattern for a period of four weeks. Then using a structured, step-wise approach, you "rebuild" that eating pattern back to a full-fledged diet with all the options and food choices that are available.

To start, you must agree to follow a defined eating pattern for four weeks. At the end of those four weeks you add one of my pre-defined categories of food into your eating regimen. I provide the list of categories and you choose which one to add in. This gives you total control over the rebuild. The starting point is a dietary baseline that could be followed for life, but is quite restrictive and is not realistic for most people long term. As you add in each food category, you will be required to think about how much of that type of food you want to "allow" or "permit" back into your daily/ weekly eating pattern. All categories do not have to be allowed back in, and you are in control over which categories you add and how much of that type of food you wish to eat.

The "Baseline Diet" is defined below; it includes a list of types of food that you start with. You eat only food from the baseline diet for the first four weeks of the rebuild. Then, at the four-week point, you add one additional food category into your eating pattern and you stick with this eating pattern for two weeks (Baseline plus One). At the end of week number six, you add in a second food category and you stick with this new eating pattern (Baseline plus Two) for another two weeks. In other words, you are allowed the baseline foods, plus one additional food category that you personally choose to add for every two weeks that you are doing the rebuild. You will continue this process of adding in one additional food category every two weeks, until you have what you feel is a satisfying, nutritious eating pattern that suits your well-thought-out preferences and meets your requirements for success.

In the end, no type of food is off limits, but every time you add in a category of food above and beyond the starting Baseline Diet platform, you do so mindful about what you are allowing into your body. This results in a structured, mindful way of choosing your new "normal" eating pattern, the eating pattern that you will refer to as your "Normal Diet" going forward.

I discuss this Dietary Rebuild process individually with each of my private patients. I want to be sure they understand the overall program, the principles involved, and the process. The Dietary Rebuild protocol puts structure to the process that every patient goes through after surgery, and does so without reverting to the Personal Persecution Program mentality, where they start with a vague idea of "normal" and are expected to utilize a mix of negative, restrictive instructions on how to avoid, minimize, and stay away from certain foods. Instead, it's a process where every patient has independent decision-making power in defining his new "normal." I also do not instruct patients to follow the rigid dieting rules that so many bariatric programs seem to mindlessly pass off as good dietary advice.

Defining your new normal diet is a critical step for you to succeed after weight-loss surgery. Remember, the goal is for you to achieve your best weight, and this means finding healthful eating habits that *you* are comfortable with, that do not result in weight regain, and allow an exercise program that you enjoy. Defining your new normal diet takes some effort, and the Dietary Rebuild is a stepwise approach for you to use in finding your best, healthful eating plan.

DIETARY REBUILD PROTOCOL

<u>Step 1:</u> This begins once you have completed the healing phase of your diet, and you're able to start back on regular food.

1. Continue to drink two quarts of calorie-free beverages daily; avoid dehydration
2. Eat three meals every day: breakfast, lunch and dinner
    a) Spend no more than 20 minutes actually eating each meal
3. Eat two snacks daily, one between breakfast/lunch and one between lunch/dinner
4. Continue vitamin and mineral supplements as directed
5. You may choose to replace one meal with a high-quality, high-protein drink
    a) During this initial Step 1 of the process, I suggest that you use the recipe for "Dr. Q's World-Famous Smoothie" as your breakfast. It's packed with nutrition and provides one quart of hydration.

Foods to Include in Step 1, Baseline:

1. Low- and moderate-starch vegetables
2. All fruits, except bananas, plantain and grapes
3. Two sources of protein: fish, meat, poultry, pork or tofu
4. Calorie-free liquids
5. Nonfat and low-fat dairy (milk, yogurt, cottage cheese, egg whites)

Add-In Categories: Food categories that will be added back into your diet as you continue through the Rebuild:

1. Whole-grain bread, cereal, pasta
2. Nuts
3. Grapes and bananas
4. High-starch vegetables
5. Beans
6. Additional sources of protein: fish, meat, poultry, pork or tofu

Foods to *avoid completely* until the Final Step in the rebuild:

1. High-sugar foods, candy, sweets
2. Deep-fried foods
3. Highly processed grain products
4. Commercial cereal, crackers, pretzels
5. Commercial sauces that contain sugar, added sweetener, or starch
6. Fruit juices, soft drinks, all drinks with added sugar
7. Alcoholic beverages

When you start this protocol, set yourself up for success. This means making sure that your home is devoid of all the food items that are not on the list above. Go through your refrigerator, pantry, wherever you store food, and throw everything that is not on the Baseline List in the trash (or give it to a neighbor). Go to the grocery store with a list of what you want in your house and buy only food items that are on your list.

One pitfall to avoid is what I call "self-processing." Examples of this include certain types of food preparation such as mashed potatoes and most forms of juicing. This self-processing makes it very easy to eat a large amount of food without feeling full. For example, when you eat an average apple, it's crunchy and bulky, it requires a lot of chewing and it's highly satisfying. If you finish one apple, you will rarely eat a second apple because you are already satisfied. If you were to juice apples you could easily turn three or four apples into juice, and drink the entire thing. Basically, you've self-processed a healthful apple into a high-sugar beverage so that you can drink fruit juice and still pretend that you're "being healthy." Do not fall into this pitfall. It's a similar type of reasoning that results in people pretending they are being healthy because they eat a salad for lunch, but when they do, they smother it in ranch dressing. I don't call this type of rationalizing cheating; I call it self-sabotage. Do your best not to sabotage yourself as you go through this process.

This Dietary Rebuild is something that you are doing for yourself. The people you live with may also benefit from the process if they choose to go through it with you. If they don't want to go through the process, that's fine, but it's important that the people you live with do not sabotage you as you go through this process.

You can identify which foods in the refrigerator and pantry are on your list and what foods are not—one method is to place a piece of green-colored tape on all of the foods that are on your list.

You can review the lists I have for each category at the back of this book and choose foods to buy from those lists. Or, you can go to some authoritative source and come up with a list of foods that follow the Dietary Rebuild protocol, i.e. a list of low-starch vegetables, a list of low-starch fruits, etc. The key is to stick with the Dietary Baseline plus only the categories that you've chosen to add in as you complete the process.

Following this protocol is not that difficult. This is a serious way to redefine your normal eating pattern after surgery, and each step in the process is important. By establishing a new normal, a new baseline for yourself, you will be forever free from your old eating habits and permanent success will be yours to enjoy.

Once you purchase your Baseline food using the guidelines provided, that is the only food that you eat for the next four weeks. If you choose to go out to eat, you can still order but eat only foods off of this list. You may, of course, go to the store whenever you want and buy more food from the Baseline List. It is important that you only consume food from the Baseline List during this first month. Feel free to use any spices or herbs that you want in order to add flavor to your food. Flavor is good, it will help you achieve satisfaction when eating, and will not result in you eating more calories.

Step 2: Go to "Baseline Plus One" for weeks five and six
After four weeks, add food from one of the Add-In Categories (only one) to your daily/weekly menu.

The list of Add-In Categories is below:

1. Whole-grain bread, cereal, pasta

2. Nuts

3. Grapes, bananas and plantain

4. High-starch vegetables

5. Beans

6. Additional sources of protein: fish, meat, poultry, pork or tofu

When you choose to add in one of these categories, think about your goals and how important it is for you to add in this category of food. Be mindful and decide how much of this category you want to eat. All of these categories are healthful foods and none will result in weight gain AS LONG AS YOU DO NOT EAT TOO MUCH!

Do not add in greasy or fried foods, sweets and desserts, whole dairy products (whole milk, butter), highly processed foods or grain products, sweetened beverages or alcohol. Stick with this new, expanded dietary menu (Baseline Plus One) for two weeks, i.e. for weeks five and six of the Rebuild.

Step 3: Go to "Baseline Plus Two" for weeks seven and eight
After six weeks, add another category of food from the list of Add-In Categories to your daily/weekly menu. Again, when you choose to add in one of these categories, be mindful how much of this type of food you want to eat. All of these categories are healthful foods that, when included in your diet in moderation, will not result in weight gain.

Still, do not add in greasy or fried foods, sweets and desserts, whole dairy products (whole milk, butter), highly processed foods or grain products, sweetened beverages or alcohol.

<u>Step 4:</u> Go to "Baseline Plus Three" for weeks nine and ten
After eight weeks, add another category of food from the list of Add-In Categories to your daily/weekly menu.

Remember, as you add in foods during your Dietary Rebuild, you want to be mindful of how often you eat this type of food, how you prepare it, and how much you decide to eat. Think about how important it is to you to add in this category of food and balance that with your goals. For example, maybe you decide to add in starchy vegetables. Think about potatoes and understand that they have a high starch content, and if you self-process them (e.g. mashed potatoes), you will be eating a food that has a very high starch content that will rapidly turn into sugar in your body. The Dietary Rebuild process is a way to consciously rebuild a healthy eating pattern, thinking through your choices each step along the way, and giving yourself time to carefully choose what you want to eat and why.

At each step in the Rebuild, you give yourself two weeks to incorporate an additional food category into your normal everyday eating pattern; you are developing new eating habits as you go. When you complete this fourth step two-week period, you will have been on the Dietary Rebuild for ten weeks. This is a relatively short time, less than three months, and you have been consciously adding in an additional category of food every two weeks for the past six weeks, or for three cycles of the Rebuild. You are choosing carefully what to include as you build your new post-surgery "Normal Diet," choosing the types of food that you like, the types of food you believe are healthful and worthwhile, and how much of these foods to eat.

You can continue this process further, adding in a category every two weeks, until you have "rebuilt" a normal eating pattern that you find satisfying. Once you complete the rebuild, you will have gone through a very thoughtful process of defining what food you want to eat on a normal daily basis. The Baseline diet that you began with includes only whole, unprocessed foods that are healthful and will not result in weight gain. The "Add-in Categories" include additional healthful foods that will not result in weight gain AS LONG AS YOU DO NOT EAT TOO MUCH! You need to listen to your body when considering how much of each food you want to eat, and where it fits into your normal eating pattern. It will tell you when you are satiated. Remember the Three-S Rule; stay within the "Satisfied" range and away from "Starved" or "Stuffed." As you complete this process you will have started to develop new eating habits, and these new habits will serve you well for the rest of your life.

A key point in this rebuild process is that you have been excluding various categories of food from your diet. You haven't been eating candy, fast food, highly processed grains, and other types of food that all have a very high likelihood of packing on the pounds. The categories of food that you've been excluding are all still "out there" in our society. But you've been focusing on incorporating additional healthful foods into your normal eating pattern each step of the way. Once you have completed this process to your satisfaction, you have rebuilt your "Normal Diet." This is what you eat, this is who you are, and it's a healthy you. Over time you will modify the amount of food, and the preparations you use, but you will be able to identify all food options as being a part of your "normal" or not.

When you decide to eat food that is outside of your normal diet, you will be consciously acknowledging that fact— "This is not part of my normal diet." Because you will immediately identify it as *not* being part of your normal, you will find it easier to consider whether you truly want to allow yourself to eat it, and you will think through *how much* of it to eat. Your normal includes all the foods that help you maintain your Best Weight. Foods outside of your normal are foods that will sabotage your weight control if you eat them in any substantial quantity. Nevertheless, those foods are "out there," and all around us. Since they are readily available, you need to consciously consider those foods and make a conscious decision as to whether you really want to eat them, and if so, how much and how often.

Final Step: Consider whether you want to add in food from the categories below that, up until now, were "off limits":
1. High-sugar foods, candy, sweets
2. Deep-fried foods
3. Highly processed grain products
    a) Commercial cereal, crackers, pretzels
4. Commercial sauces that contain sugar, added sweetener, or starch
5. Fruit juices, soft drinks, all drinks with added sugar
6. Alcoholic beverages

This is a very important step; these foods are available to you and will always be. However, these categories are not a necessary part of a healthy existence. These foods are truly optional; there is nothing, NOTHING, about food from any of these categories that is required to make you healthier. These foods are highly addicting, cause medical diseases, and can rapidly result in weight gain. You just spent well over three months not eating any of these foods, and you are succeeding in long-term weight control, you are improving your health, you are increasing your range of capability, and your quality of life is improving. So, be careful and really think about whether it is worth adding this stuff into your diet, and if so, how often and how much.

These "Final Step" food categories are not part of your Normal Diet. However, I know of many healthy-weight people that eat foods from all of these categories ONCE IN A WHILE, and IN LIMITED QUANTITY. I do not know of any truly fit people (other than an occasional intense athlete) who eat these foods often. When people begin to eat these foods in any significant quantity THEY GAIN WEIGHT.

You don't have to allow these Final Step foods back into your diet, but if you do, think about how much and how often. Think about your goals and how important it is for you to add in this category of food. No category of foods is absolutely off-limits, but know that there is a price, in terms of your weight, your health, and your quality of life, that you will pay if you choose to eat very much of these foods.

Once you finish this Dietary Rebuild process you will have a personally defined eating pattern that enables you to maintain your desired level of fitness and health. You will have identified a new "Normal" diet that allows you to maintain your BEST WEIGHT, forever.

EXERCISE HABITS

In addition to developing new eating habits, the other lifestyle improvement that is critical in achieving permanent success with weight-loss surgery is exercise. It's an acknowledged fact among most weight-loss experts that eating fewer calories is what enables you to lose weight, but these experts also know that *exercise is required* to complete the process.

Now before you throw this book down, stomp on it and yell, "But I don't like to exercise!" just take a deep breath and remember that the very reason you are reading this book is because you want to be able to do more in life, you want to participate fully, you want to be more *fit*. Exercise is a key step in achieving that goal, and if you approach exercise the right way, you'll find that you enjoy it. In this chapter I go into what exercise really means and why everyone that does it enjoys it.

As I discussed early in this book, the real goal of patients seeking weight-loss surgery is *not* really weight loss. The real goal is to be able to do the things that you currently feel uncomfortable doing, or you simply can't do, with all the excess body fat. In other words, the reason you are looking into weight loss is to be able to increase your ability to do things, or to "increase your range of capability."

> "My friends and I enjoy kayaking now, and I'm always looking for new things to try that I would never have been able to do being overweight. Caring for my two precious grandchildren is so much easier now, with my new mobility and energy level. Getting up from the floor is no longer burdensome, and I can actually play with them now and participate in life!"
>
> **Cheryl B.**
> **Preschool Teacher**

Remember your goal to expand your range of capability. So the real goal, once again, is to improve your fitness, and this means exercise. Exercise may be outside of your comfort zone but, guess what, your *entire goal* is to do things that are currently outside of your comfort zone! So, you now have a choice: decide that you are sadly mistaken and you really don't want to improve your fitness, grab the remote control, hit the couch, and forget about permanent weight loss. Or, you can accept that the things you are dying to do, the things you believe are fun, actually involve some exercise.

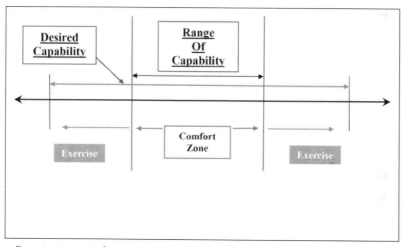

Exercise is required to increase your "Range of Capability" (your Comfort Zone)

"I now celebrate November 26th each year. This was my surgery date. I celebrate this day as much as my actual birthday because this is when I began my new life! Today I have lost over half my body weight. I weigh 175 pounds and have never been happier. About four months after my surgery I discovered how it felt to walk to the top of the stairs without losing my breath. By six months after surgery I was trying things that I never would have even dreamed of in my old life. I had taken up surfing, playing tennis and running. I ran my first 5K September of 2008! I run races regularly now. My life has turned around."

Michelle G.

Payroll Manager

People often ask why exercise alone cannot result in substantial, permanent weight loss. First, think about how easily you can eat more than 1,000 calories. One serving of the crispy chicken tenders at McDonald's is 500 calories, a Caramel Frappuccino® and blueberry scone at Starbucks comes to 800 calories, and one breakfast burrito at The Cheesecake Factory gives you over 2,500 calories. Now, consider that if you continuously perform *intense* exercise, such as running or mountain biking, non-stop for an entire hour, you will burn off less than 1,000 calories. Simply walking as fast as you can, at about three miles per hour, will only burn off between 100 and 150 calories per mile. In other words, unless you're an athlete and can perform extreme exercise for hours on end, it could take days to burn off the calories you can consume in a single high-calorie sitting. And an hour a day of exercise is certainly not enough to overcome twenty-three hours a day of bad eating habits.

Knowing that you started this process specifically in order to be able to feel better and do more physically, the only question is, "Will you?" As I'm writing this portion of the book, I just discharged seven people from the hospital less than twenty-four hours after their surgery, and I am ecstatic to say that five of those seven patients specifically asked me, "When will I be healed enough that can I start exercising?"

I love that question!! I love it because almost every patient comes into my office believing that they want to lose weight "for my health" and saying things like, "Losing weight will improve my blood pressure." And, as I do with EVERY one of my patients during their first consultation, I discuss their activity level and by the end of the discussion they are saying, "That's so true, I really can't do what I want to do with all this weight, and YES, my main goal is that I want to *do* more!" And then they commit to fitness and exercise as part of their weight-loss process. So, it's incredibly gratifying to me when patients truly have this understanding and commitment, and are so on-target with the concept of fitness after their surgery has been completed.

GET STARTED ON YOUR PERSONAL EXERCISE PROGRAM

You have already had the surgery and are losing weight and developing new eating habits, so beginning an exercise program is the second key part of the process for success.

First Step: Identify Initial Goals
Take a few minutes to sit down and think about activities that you would like to do on a regular basis, but that you struggle with or simply can't do. Write down two or three activities that come up on a daily or weekly basis in your life, that you would like to be able to do that you couldn't do before. These might be exciting things,

but more often they are things that you want to be able to do that are simple, common and are part of a normal daily life. These few things should be activities that you would love to be able to do without having to think about it.

Examples of things that my patients list:

- Be able to walk the entire shopping mall without having to sit down to rest
- Practice kicking a soccer ball with your daughter or son
- Go hiking in the local hills on Saturdays
- Join your friend in her weekly yoga class
- Go dancing with your wife or husband
- Play on a local softball team

Some of my patients are young and active and are able to do everything on this list already, but they want to do more. I have patients that are very active, despite their obesity, but want to be able to run a 10K without feeling like their ankles are going to break. Other patients only dream of doing the things listed above despite only being in their twenties or thirties, because their weight causes so much pain and damage already. Everyone has a different threshold for deciding that "enough is enough" with their excess weight and that, "now is the time to do something about it."

It does not matter what your threshold is, what matters is that you've hit your limit and you've decided that increasing your range of capability is an absolute must. So, whatever these things are that you want to do, *now* is the time to sit down and acknowledge them. You don't need to list them all, but a short list of significant things that you would like to do on a daily/weekly basis will help get you started and serve as a useful point of reference in the future.

One caveat: this list should include only activities that require action, not activities that require no movement. Examples of actions that require no movement, but that my patients often mention include 1) sit comfortably on an airplane, 2) sit comfortably in a booth in a restaurant, 3) be able to sit comfortably on rides in the local amusement park. All of these activities may be important, but they involve little or no movement. Thinking only about these things will not help you succeed. For example, if the airplane built wider seats, the restaurant had bigger booths, or the amusement park retrofitted their rides to hold morbidly obese people, then none of these things would be meaningful. As long as they keep building bigger booths, bigger seats and bigger scooters, you'll be able to simply get fatter and fatter while the world accommodates your size. Clearly, this is not the goal here, so when making your list of daily/weekly activities, stick with things that require physical action.

Second Step: Use this list, and the ROC Graph, to plan your initial exercise program.

Take one activity that you want to be able to do and mark a place for it on the Range of Capability graph. (Since this is a "Want-To," it will be *outside* of your current Range of Capability.) Once you place a mark for this activity (e.g. go hiking in the local hills), write down a physical activity that you think you *are* currently capable of doing that is similar to this particular Want-To, but that you "Can-Do" now (e.g. walk around the block). Now mark a place for this "Can-Do" activity on your ROC graph. (This mark will be *inside* your Range of Capability.) Now, you have a diagram that shows you in a graphic way the difference between something you are capable of doing now, and something you *want* to be able to do.

Planning how to get from your Can-Do-Now to your Want-To involves two things: the first is to set up a *schedule* where you are going to do this activity, or exercise, on a regular basis (the best is daily), and the second is to decide *when* to begin (now is usually the best answer). For the example above, where hiking in the hills is your Want-To and being able to walk around the block is your Can-Do-Now, a good plan would be to start by walking around the block every day for one week, then increase the distance every week, until you are fit enough to begin short hikes in the hills. In other words, methodically bridge the gap between Can-Do-Now and Want-To.

Examples from my patients:

1. Jim had been a distance runner and soccer player in high school, but at 46 years old he had spent most of the past 30 years focusing on work and his children's needs. At 5'8" and 250 pounds, he was 110 pounds over his high school running weight, had bad knees and chronic back pain, and jogging was a distant fantasy. Nevertheless, he often thought of joining the community soccer league. He lost 10 pounds with his pre-operative diet and another 20 at four weeks after surgery. With his 30-pound weight loss, he found that he no longer got short of breath walking in the neighborhood, so he expanded his daily walking program. He committed to get up 45 minutes early and do a half-hour walk before taking his shower and heading to work. He was worried about aggravating his joint pain so he started conservatively, initially walking one mile. The going was slow at first since he was still overweight, but he was able to do it. He didn't succeed with walking every single day, but he made certain to walk at least five days a week. As he continued, he began to feel stronger, and as his weight continued to

decrease, he felt lighter on his feet. After four weeks he added another mile. He had to walk faster with the extra distance in order to keep the total exercise time down around 30 minutes, and at two miles he was walking very fast. He continued this for another three months, until about six months after surgery, and by then he had lost a total of 80 pounds. He was now 5'8" and 170 pounds. At six months after surgery, he bought some running shoes and began to do a slow jog. Jim stayed consistent with his plan and even took up jogging again as a hobby. He decided that he didn't really have the time to join the soccer league, but he now runs in three or four 5K races each year. He never achieved his high school weight of 140 pounds, but his weight has stayed at about 155 pounds for the past seven years.

2. Kathy, at 62, was 5'8" and 280 pounds, 140 pounds *over* her ideal body weight. She was widowed, her children were grown and had families of their own, and she was very successful in business, but she had no social life other than at work. After surgery, she joined a gym and did water aerobics classes but these just didn't do it for her. At one of her follow-up appointments we discussed her exercise and she said she wasn't thrilled with it. She was down 40 pounds at three months, but didn't feel motivated. During our conversation, she told me that her late husband and she had loved to ballroom dance. I suggested that she join a dance school and take some lessons, get her skills back. Kathy signed up at a commercial dance school and began lessons twice a week. She loved it. She also found that instead of water aerobics she was able to start regular aerobics classes. These involved similar movements to some of her ballroom dancing and she felt this made her ballroom skills better. She increased

her aerobics classes to three days a week and continued her ball-room dancing at two or three days every week. To my satisfaction, Kathy actually got down to her ideal body weight. She had some extra skin, and used some of her savings for a tummy tuck and breast lift and after all this she looked great! She started dating men that she met ballroom dancing, and even entered some dancing competitions. Kathy kept her weight off and remained active the rest of her life, passing away at 80 years of age.

Both of these patients started with an activity they could do, a Can-Do-Now, and eventually were capable of their Want-To, even exceeding their fitness goals. If it weren't for the weight loss they achieved through surgery and the exercise plan *they stuck to*, these dreams would never have become a reality.

Below is the Range of Capability Graph with an example for identifying a Can-Do-Now and a Want-To. Start with one or two of these, and get going.

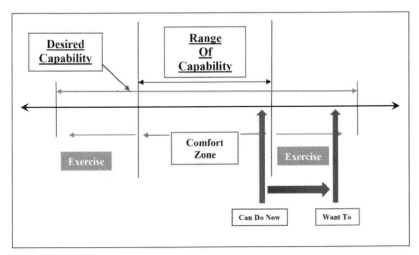

"Range of Capability": Starting Your Exercise Program

I asked a successful patient the following question, five years after surgery: "Your thoughts on obesity, now that you have succeeded with weight loss?"

His answer:

"It (was) a HORRIBLE place to be, and NO one who has never been there can know what it is like. It is totally an alone feeling that is hard to beat, but it is NOT unbeatable! You have to take charge, listen to your desire to be healthy and know that this will give you a leg up. Keep in mind, the surgery is a surgical procedure NOT a magical procedure! You still have to do your part. You have to embrace exercise, embrace good food and healthy living!"

Joe K.
Regional Sales Manager

TOOLS

Below is a tool you might find useful in coming up with a reasonable starting point. Create a small worksheet on a single piece of paper using the process below.

1. Ask yourself, "Was I ever an athlete?" This is a Yes or No. If the answer is Yes, then write down the last age at which you truly were still competing in that sport.

   a) First, if you were never an athlete, that's not a bad thing. It doesn't mean that you can never become an athlete, but it may be possible that athletics is just not your bag. If it isn't your thing, then having a goal of becoming an athlete will be counterproductive. You can still develop a very healthful exercise program without the expectation of becoming an athlete, and you can enjoy physical activity that isn't a sport. (Kathy's goal of ballroom dancing is an example.)

b) If you were an athlete, then take note of when that was. If you're 55 years old, the fact that you were a star soccer player in high school doesn't mean that your goal should be to win the city league soccer championship. However, like Jim, above, you can still increase your capability to a level where you are happy with what you are capable of doing.

c) Writing down the maximum capability you have achieved in life, and when that was, helps to put things in perspective and might help you identify a goal that you can achieve.

Regardless of how you define it, you need a goal. In other words:

> *"If your goal is nothing, you're bound to achieve it."*
> - **Brian Quebbemann, M.D.**

A WORD OF CAUTION

There are many ways to succeed but there are also many ways to fail. You will fail if you never start, if you quit, or if you go back into denial and tell yourself that it's all OK to be obese. But, there are also ways to fail that are not so obvious.

Below I list three patterns of fitness failure that I've seen in my practice. None of them are due to laziness or lack of commitment. Rather, they are due to an overzealous ambition, resulting in self-defeat. I hate it when I see these, because the people that fail as a result of goals that are too lofty are patients who were very committed but just sabotaged themselves with over-intensity. Some of them have regrouped and started a more reasonable fitness program, but some of them became upset that their goals were excessive and then quit altogether rather than accept a more reasonable plan.

PATTERNS OF FITNESS FAILURE

Avoid these:

1. Extreme goals resulting in self-defeat
   a) This is where a patient gets it into their head that they "should" be able to do something, without thinking, "Is this really in the realm of possibility?"
   b) Remember, it's better to start with something you know is achievable, and then elevate your goals over time.

2. Excessive intensity resulting in injury, downtime and exercise resentment
   a) This occurs when someone simply tries to get where they're going too fast.
   b) This is a process. It didn't take you six months to get out of shape and it's unlikely that you'll become fit in six months.
   c) You're setting yourself up for a lifelong level of fitness. Take your time, do it right.

3. All Pain for Gain

a) This is where you choose something you actually don't like to do at all, usually because "it's good for me" or you believe that you *should* like it.

b) I see this with people who base their goals on what someone else, a friend, family member, neighbor, is capable of doing instead of what they really think they want to do.

OK, I've talked a lot about fitness versus weight loss, about range of capability, and about how to begin on a self-defined exercise program that will bring you to the level of fitness you want. Now, get on with it.

INTERVIEW WITH A SUCCESSFUL PATIENT

Interviewer: You exercise regularly now; do you think that modifies how you eat?

Kim: Oh, my goodness. Oh, boy where do I even start with that? Endorphins, muscle mass –

Interviewer: Well, think about timing. If you're gonna go and exercise, do you put down a banana split beforehand?

Kim: No, because – once you change your obsession, it's all about the workout and you get up in the morning and you eat so you can have a good workout.

Interviewer: Why do you want a good workout? What about it is good? Do you feel good afterwards or what?

Kim: Yes, for me it's stress reduction and discipline.

Interviewer: Don't tell me you do workouts because you enjoy discipline?

Kim: I do, I do. Isn't that crazy?

Interviewer: No, it's not. You enjoy workouts because you like the routine?

Kim: The routine, yeah, just doing what I say I'm gonna do when I say I'm gonna do it.

Interviewer: Okay, so it's self-fulfilling?

Kim: Yeah– gosh, I said I was gonna go three times and I went three times.

Interviewer: Okay, for you it's like "Check box checked, I won this week"?

Kim: Yeah, it means I managed all the revolving pieces so I could actually do what I said I was gonna do.

Interviewer: Okay, so the exercise kind of reinforces the fact that you –

Kim: – You have control.

Interviewer: Yeah, you're in control and you're doing something for yourself.

Kim: Yeah, and I think you said it in your clinic, that you start to treat yourself equal to everybody else instead of "less than." In the past it's like you make sure everybody else gets where they're supposed to go and then you don't. But treating yourself as an equal is a brilliant concept, rather than treating yourself as a "less than."

Interviewer: Yeah, that's a hard one though. That's a hard one to overcome.

Kim: You don't have to be better than others. It doesn't mean that you're "better than." It means you're just the same as.

Interviewer: Yeah, it means you respect yourself. Is exercise a manifestation of respecting yourself then?

Kim: Yeah, it's great, the endorphins and the accomplishment and the positive feedback and the camaraderie.

SECTION 5:

ADDITIONAL INFORMATION

BRIEF OVERVIEW OF METABOLIC SURGERY

Putting the word "cure" into the management of obesity-induced metabolic disease.

Obesity-induced metabolic diseases are traditionally thought of as *treatable*, but not as *curable*, and the medications used to treat these conditions are required for life. Physicians have aggressively treated obesity-induced metabolic diseases such as diabetes with reasonable results. Other obesity-induced metabolic diseases, in particular severe obesity, have historically suffered from a complete failure of medical intervention to produce a safe and effective treatment.

Long-term weight loss and improved fitness can result in the dramatic improvement of obesity-induced metabolic disease. Unfortunately, the only "cures" have been with the rare individuals that have lost most of their excess weight and kept it off by succeeding in major lifestyle change, effectively curing themselves. The medical treatments for obesity-induced metabolic diseases, however, have never provided a "cure."

The Cost of Obesity-induced Metabolic Disease
Medications required to treat obesity-induced metabolic diseases

are very expensive and add up to considerable sums over a lifetime. The annual direct cost of treating the 67 million Americans (CDC, 2011) with hypertension was estimated at $47.5 billion, or about $710 per patient, adding up to more than $21,000 over 30 years. This $21,000 does not take into account the cost of side effects of the medications, nor does it account for all those additional diseases, such as kidney failure, stroke and heart disease, that develop as a result of long-standing hypertension.

Direct medical costs for treating the more than 25 million Americans (CDC, 2011) with diabetes is estimated at $176 billion, or $6,800 annually per patient, or over $200,000 per patient over 30 years. And, as a leading cause for stroke, heart failure, heart attack, kidney disease, blindness and amputation, the overall cost of diabetes adds up quickly. Other obesity-induced metabolic diseases carry a high cost as well, not only in terms of medical treatment, but also in terms of missed work, lost wages and human suffering.

Taken as a group, obesity-induced metabolic disease adds huge costs to our healthcare system and exacts an immeasurable toll on our society in terms of lost productivity and patient suffering.

The Role for Surgery

Metabolic surgery is the specialty of surgery that addresses obesity-induced metabolic disease as potentially curable. Historically, metabolic surgery has mainly focused on severe obesity and operations have been primarily targeted towards weight loss. The first reason for this was that severe obesity is highly recalcitrant to all other medical intervention, being difficult to treat and nearly impossible to cure. The second reason was that the impact of these operations on long-term weight loss was dramatic and easy to document. Over the past three decades, however, it has become increasingly apparent that the operations used for weight loss have a significant positive impact on several other metabolic disorders. In fact, the success with resolving hypertension, hyperlipidemia and Type II diabetes through weight-loss surgery has resulted in new areas of research on the role of the gastrointestinal tract in the management of metabolic disease.

The most exciting clinical revelation has been that performing gastrointestinal surgery to treat obesity-induced metabolic disease can, in fact, result in a cure. The potential for metabolic operations to actually cure these diseases is now an irrefutable fact, and has resulted in a paradigm shift where certain obesity-induced metabolic diseases are no longer considered to be lifelong illnesses.

Published in the *Journal of the American Medical Association* in 2004, a meta-analysis of 22,049 patients that had undergone traditional bariatric surgery showed an overall 61% sustained excess body weight loss. In terms of obesity-induced metabolic disease the study showed a 76.8% resolution of Type II diabetes, a 61.7% resolution of hypertension, and a 79.3% improvement in hyperlipidemia. In a more recent study examining 23,000 patients with metabolic syndrome that underwent bariatric surgery, 36%, 50% and 35% had complete remission of hypertension, diabetes and dyslipidemia, respectively.

Successful resolution of obesity-induced metabolic disease after metabolic surgery is far from 100%. Nevertheless, the fact that diseases previously thought of as only treatable are now known to be potentially curable is incredibly important. Patients suffering from these disease processes, when caused by obesity, can now be counseled that there is an opportunity for cure. In fact, in my professional opinion, if a patient meets the criteria for metabolic surgical therapy, it is now below the standard of care for a physician counseling that patient to fail to make them aware of the possibility for surgical treatment of their disease.

Who Qualifies for Metabolic Surgery?

The National Institutes of Health (NIH) published guidelines for bariatric surgery after a 1991 consensus conference. These guidelines are currently published on their website with a disclaimer (reprinted below) stating that the guidelines are outdated. Despite advancements over the past 25 years resulting in safer bariatric procedures (decreased risk) and a higher level of success (improved benefit), Medicare and commercial insurers have refused to update the guidelines and still refer to the 1991 guidelines when authorizing payment for these surgeries.

The 1991 NIH guidelines were based on an extensive benefit-versus-risk analysis, and are fairly simple:

"Patients whose BMI exceeds 40 are potential candidates for surgery if they strongly desire substantial weight loss, because obesity severely impairs the quality of their lives. In certain instances less severely obese patients (with BMI's between 35 and 40) also may be considered for surgery. Included in this category are patients with high-risk comorbid conditions and patients with obesity-induced physical problems interfering with lifestyle (e.g., joint disease treatable but for the obesity, or body size problems precluding or severely interfering with employment, family function, and ambulation)."

Following these 1991 guidelines, the insurance industry will generally authorize patients to undergo bariatric surgery if they have a BMI>40, or a BMI = 35-40 with significant weight-related disease or disability.

More up-to-date indications for metabolic surgery have been published, and provide reasonable guidelines for when to consider surgery. These modern guidelines take into account the preponderance of scientific data showing that most patients with a BMI of 30 or greater have a markedly increased risk for obesity-induced diseases including diabetes, heart disease, cancer and physical disability. They also take into account the lack of adequate alternative treatments for obesity. In fact, the health risks for a BMI of 30 or greater (defined medically as the threshold for obesity) is so well accepted that the FDA approved the Lap-Band device for treating patients with a BMI as low as 30.

From the published statement on the FDA website (updated 9/6/2013)

"The LAP-BAND® System is used for weight loss in obese adults who have a Body Mass Index(BMI) of 30-40, with one or more obesity-related medical conditions (such as Type II diabetes and hypertension), and when non-surgical weight loss methods (such as supervised diet, exercise, and behavior modification) have not been successful."

The take-home message is that, based on the safety and success of modern metabolic surgical procedures, it is reasonable to offer weight-loss surgery for any patient with a BMI>35, and all individuals with a BMI between 30 and 35 who have failed at long-term weight loss and complain of a significantly decreased quality of life or who suffer from weight-related medical disease.

The disclaimer from the National Institutes of Health pertaining to the lack of updated published indications for metabolic surgery is reprinted below.

Disclaimer on the NIH website:

http://consensus.nih.gov/1991/1991gisurgeryobesity084html.htm

> "This statement is more than five years old and is provided solely for historical purposes. Due to the cumulative nature of medical research, new knowledge has inevitably accumulated in this subject area in the time since the statement was initially prepared. Thus some of the material is likely to be out of date, and at worst simply wrong."

It's unfortunate that a national agency is unwilling to update its published guidelines on such a widespread disease. The only explanations I can come up with are that there is a concern that up-to-date guidelines would result in an increased demand for weight-loss surgery, or simply that ignoring the plight of obese people is still an acceptable bias in our society. The good news is that individual experts and professional organizations have updated their guidelines over time.

Education: The First Step in the Metabolic Surgery Process
The first step in the metabolic surgery process is education of the patient, and a reality check. Metabolic surgery has a high degree of success, and if done correctly has a low surgical risk. However, like most medical treatments, compliance on the part of the patient is

key to obtaining the best result. And, because the only reasonable goal for someone undergoing metabolic surgery is to achieve long-term or permanent success, up-front understanding of the patient role in the surgical treatment process is mandatory.

All patients need to be advised that maximum long-term success is dependent on lifestyle changes that they should find to be far easier to achieve with the help provided through surgery. However, these changes need to be desired and truly pursued if they are to become a reality in a patient's life. All patients need to have it clear in their minds that, for long-term success, healthful changes in eating behavior need to be embraced. Healthful eating takes understanding and effort whether a person has been overweight or not, and only those patients who use the surgical procedure to assist them in improving their diet will succeed. In fact, the scientific literature is fairly clear on the fact that long-term success is also dependent on patients embracing a physically active lifestyle, including daily exercise. Studies have shown that the surgical patients who use their surgery to achieve a healthy lifestyle can obtain permanent weight loss, dramatic metabolic improvement, and an improved quality of life. Only through patient compliance are the risks of surgery justified by the dramatic benefits achieved.

What are the Standard Metabolic Surgical Procedures?
Bypass Operations:
A very brief history of bariatric surgery begins more than 60 years ago, in 1953, with Dr. Victor Henrikson of Gothenburg, Sweden who performed an intestinal resection to treat obesity, and Dr. Richard Varco, at the University of Minnesota, who performed the world's first intestinal bypass to treat obesity. For the next 25 years, operations for obesity consisted primarily of malabsorption oper-

ations, specifically various kinds of intestinal bypasses, the jejuno-ileal bypass being the most common. These operations resulted in a high degree of malnutrition and fell out of favor more than 30 years ago. In 1967 a less malabsorptive operation, the gastric bypass, was invented by Dr. Edward E. Mason at the University of Iowa, and this operation has been improved over the last 50 years to the current laparoscopic gastric bypass which is still considered to be the gold-standard bariatric operation. Around 1980, the gastric bypass was changed to the Roux-en-Y Gastric bypass, and this minimized the symptoms of GERD and heartburn which had been experienced with the initial procedure. However, as a result of the complications seen with intestinal bypass, the term "bypass" came to falsely represent operations with a high risk of severe malnutrition. The gastric bypass involves only a limited intestinal bypass, mainly bypassing the stomach, whereas operations that carry a higher risk for malnutrition are those that involve bypass of a substantial portion of small intestine. Two operations that involve substantial intestinal bypass, the Biliopancreatic Diversion (BPD) introduced by Dr. Nicola Scopinaro in 1979 at the University of Genoa, Italy, and the Duodenal Switch (DS) designed by Dr. Douglas Hess of Ohio in 1986, are still performed by some surgeons. The BPD and DS operations are remarkably effective operations for treating diabetes and severe dyslipidemia (high cholesterol and high triglycerides), but carry with them a high risk for malnutrition.

Restrictive Operations:
Around 1979 Dr. Mason also invented the gastroplasty, which carried no risk for malabsorption and was called a "restrictive operation" because it forced patients to eat slowly and chew well. Various forms of gastroplasty (also called "stomach stapling")

were used for about 20 years but, despite successful weight loss, the complications including chronic vomiting were high and the operation fell out of favor. In the late 1990s gastric banding was started in Europe and eventually converted to an adjustable gastric band procedure. Then in 2001 the FDA approved a laparoscopic adjustable gastric band procedure, the Lap-Band System™, for use in the United States. The Lap-Band turned out to be a very safe operation, and surged in popularity for more than ten years, but its popularity has declined due to bad press from Lap-Band centers that had multiple complications and also from the introduction of a newer restrictive operation with better results, the Vertical Sleeve Gastrectomy (VSG, or Sleeve). The "Sleeve" procedure has weight loss comparable to the gastric bypass, but with no intestinal bypass so the risk of malabsorption is minimal.

Currently, the most common operations in the world are the sleeve gastrectomy, the gastric bypass and the lap-band, all performed using minimally invasive surgery (laparoscopy). The graph below demonstrates some of the differences between these operations. (Data specific to Dr. Quebbemann.)

Procedure	Gastric bypass	Sleeve Gastrectomy	Lap-Band
Average Length of Operation	50-60 minutes	30-45 minutes	30-45 minutes
Typical Hospital Stay	1 day	Outpatient-to-1 day	Outpatient
Average Weight Loss	70% of excess (40-100%)	65% of excess (40-100%)	50% of excess (0-100%)
Significant Nutritional Issues	Uncommon	Rare	Rare
Nutritional Supplements	Highly Recommended	Highly Recommended	Recommended
Reversibility	Yes	No	Yes

Observations on Metabolic Surgery and Future Directions

Although it may seem like the positive effect metabolic surgery has on diabetes, hypertension and other disease is a recent discovery, the fact is that the use of surgery to treat obesity-induced metabolic diseases was being studied in the 1960s. As the evidence grew for surgery as a primary treatment for high cholesterol, high triglycerides and Type II diabetes in obese patients, the physiologic effects of the different operations began to be more closely examined. Due in part to the dramatic improvement in diabetes after gastric bypass, and the dramatic improvement in hyperlipidemia after intestinal bypass, the important role of hormones produced by the stomach and small intestine in the regulation of insulin, blood sugar and metabolism has become apparent. These observations have now culminated in intensive research into the use of surgery specifically to treat obesity-induced metabolic disease, particularly as a treatment for diabetes.

In September 2008 the first World Congress on Interventional Therapies for Type II Diabetes was held in New York. The excitement at this meeting focused on evidence that surgery could be performed safely, on non-obese individuals, specifically to resolve diabetes without weight loss. Interest in these concepts resulted in studies on surgical procedures to treat Type II diabetes being conducted throughout the world.

With an improved understanding of the role of the gastrointestinal tract, and its importance in controlling cholesterol, triglycerides, insulin and our metabolism in general, the field of metabolic surgery is evolving. It is now very important for all physicians to understand modern metabolic surgery and its role as a treatment for obesity-induced metabolic disease, and sometimes as a cure.

References

Buchwald H, Varco RL. Ileal bypass in lowering high cholesterol levels. Surg Forum 1964; 15:289-291

Buchwald H, Varco RL. lleal bypass in patients with hypercholesterolemia and atherosclerosis: Preliminary report on therapeutic potential. JAMA 1966; 196:627-630

Pories WJ. Why does the gastric bypass control Type II diabetes mellitus? *Obes Surg.* 1992; 2:303–313

Forgacs S, Halmos T. Improvement of glucose tolerance in diabetics following gastrectomy [in German]. *Z Gastroenterol.* 1973; 11:293–296

Steven Grover S, et al. Preventing cardiovascular disease among Canadians: Is the treatment of hypertension or dyslipidemia cost-effective? Can J Cardiol 2008; 24(12):891-898

Inabnet WB, et al. Early Outcomes of Bariatric Surgery in Patients with Metabolic Syndrome: An Analysis of the Bariatric Outcomes Longitudinal Database. J Am Coll Surg, 2012, 214, (4):556-557

Bariatric surgery in class 1 obesity (body mass index 30-35 kg/m2), ASMBS statements/guidelines, September 12, 2012

Buchwald H, et al. Bariatric Surgery, A Systematic Review and Meta-analysis. JAMA. 2004; 292:1724-1737

Raul J. Rosenthal, M.D., F.A.C.S., F.A.S.M.B.S.*, for the International Sleeve Gastrectomy Expert Panel Consensus Statement. Surgery for Obesity and Related Diseases 8 (2012) 8 –19

GENERAL COMMENTS ON THE BAND, SLEEVE AND BYPASS

1. All bariatric operations are complex. The surgeon needs to perform the operation in a way that results, in the end, in very specific anatomy. In other words, if the anatomy of the stomach and intestine is not correct at the end of the operation, the operation will not work. This is not always easy to do since every person is shaped differently inside (just like we all are shaped differently on the outside). The surgeon must be focused on performing the operation correctly in order to give his or her patients the best chance for success.

2. If you eat high-calorie soft foods, or high-calorie liquids, you will be able to take in a lot of calories without feeling full. This is a way to minimize the beneficial effects of the Gastric Sleeve, the Gastric Band and the Gastric Bypass. I call this "SABOTAGE" because it means that you've chosen to undergo an operation to help you eat slowly and modify your eating pattern, and then you've figured out how to "get around" the operation. Most patients do not sabotage themselves, and as a result, they succeed in modifying their diet and losing a substantial amount of weight.

3. The speed of the operation is not a main goal; although novice surgeons may think that speed makes them "better" this is NOT

TRUE. The important goal with these operations (and all surgery) is to get the operation done correctly, and to have a low complication rate. Nothing else is important. Bariatric surgeons must focus on getting the operation done correctly, and in the safest way possible.

Technical Addenda

PRE-AND POST-OPERATIVE TESTING PROTOCOLS

Pre-operative testing is mandatory prior to bariatric surgery in order to reduce the risk of complications. Bariatric surgery patients carry a higher surgical risk secondary to their obesity and the multiple comorbid medical conditions that accompany severe obesity. My goal at The N.E.W. Program has been to successfully maximize patient safety through reasonable evidence-based protocols. All studies ordered at The N.E.W. Program are for the benefit of the patient. We do not maximize the number of tests ordered, in fact we have always tried to minimize the number of tests in order to avoid inconvenience to our patients. However, a thorough evaluation and appropriate testing has always been a mandatory part of our pre-operative and post-op process.

All tests we order at baseline prior to surgery also provide a baseline for future post-operative comparison to monitor our patient's progress. Below is a list of the testing that may be ordered on our patients to ensure safety and success with their bariatric surgery. Testing ordered by our specialists is based on each patient's unique situation. Tests highlighted BOLD BLACK are required in every case. Tests in BOLD BACK UNDERLINE are commonly ordered, but not in every case. Other less common tests are also listed.

The list below is not comprehensive, and additional testing will be done as needed.

Laboratory Blood Testing is required and my basic bariatric surgery blood test panel is shown on the following pages. Almost every pre-surgical patient has some form of malnutrition, although most are minor, and we base our recommendations for supplementation in part on the results of these tests. Other tests often identify diseases that patients may not know they have, such as high cholesterol or diabetes.

EKG or "echocardiogram" is obtained for all patients as the standard test that demonstrates the normal electrical rhythm of his or her heart. If indicated, additional testing and referral to a cardiologist are required.

Chest X-Ray is required before surgery to demonstrate normal heart and lung anatomy.

Abdominal Ultrasound is obtained due to the extremely high prevalence of obesity-induced liver damage seen prior to bariatric surgery. This test is used to assess liver size (which can affect surgical safety), degree of fatty infiltration of the liver (non-alcoholic fatty liver disease, NAFLD) as well as the presence of damage to the liver by excess body fat (NASH or cirrhosis). It also assesses for gallstones. Due to the post-operative anatomy, presence of gall-stones is highly significant. In addition, symptoms of gallbladder disease can mimic complications of bariatric surgery, or even adversely modify a patient's diet.

Spirometry is done to assess pulmonary function. This can be important prior to general anesthesia. When this test is significantly abnormal, referral to a pulmonologist is considered.

Upper Endoscopy is often done to evaluate patients with GERD or heartburn. Hiatal hernia, found in a large of percentage of patients with GERD, is typically repaired at the time of their bariatric procedure.

Upper GI X-ray is also done to assess patients with GERD or heartburn. This test provides a picture of the esophageal and gastric anatomy.

Resting Metabolic Rate can be very helpful when counseling patients concerning metabolism, diet and exercise. RMR can help to monitor metabolic improvement seen with decreased body fat and improved muscle tone due to exercise. This test also helps evaluate patients who are not losing weight effectively.

Body Composition is, in my opinion, more important than patient weight. Lean muscle mass and body fat ratio affects hormone balance and metabolism. It also helps to determine risk for heart disease.

Sleep Study is used to evaluate patients with signs or symptoms of sleep apnea. Sleep apnea can affect the safety of general anesthesia, and untreated sleep apnea can adversely affect a patient's energy level and ability to exercise.

Bone Density Scan looks for early bone loss and osteoporosis, both of which are found at a higher incidence in obese individuals.

Lower Extremity Ultrasound is done to assess for deep venous thrombosis (DVT, blood clots) in patients with significant leg swelling, or a history of prior DVT, and sometimes for other indications such as calf tenderness.

Thyroid Ultrasound is done on all patients with thyroid abnormalities on physical examination or history of thyroid disease that is poorly controlled.

Basic Nutritional Guidelines

Guidelines in Place of Rules

1. Eat Chewable Food, Not "Mush".
Chewing food provides more satisfaction when eating. Also, adequate chewing is important to avoid discomfort after bariatric surgery.

Eating soft, mushy foods that do not require chewing will decrease your satisfaction, resulting in less satiety and the need to eat a larger volume of food, and thereby limit your success. (Mac and cheese and mashed potatoes are examples of high-calorie mush.)

2. Eat two to three meals per day and at least two snacks per day.
Eating regularly during the day will maintain a higher metabolism. Skipping meals will also result in fluctuations of your blood sugar and energy level and may result in cravings and headaches.

Always eat something for breakfast (in a pinch, a high-protein smoothie is a good substitute).

3. At least three of your meals per day should be high-protein meals.
Remember "protein first." This expression is used not because protein has been proven to be the most important food group, but because a balanced diet is important. Protein is required for healthy muscle development and results in more satiety than carbohydrates. When eating smaller portions, following a pattern of starting with protein-based foods (meat, fish, tofu, eggs) will help

to ensure balanced nutrition. Protein seems to be the easiest food group to skimp on, and most of my patients are used to eating too many refined carbohydrates (cereal, chips, tortillas, pasta) and far too little protein.

4. Drink at least two quarts of calorie-free beverages per day. Drink one glass of water, 15-30 minutes prior to regular meals. Minimize drinking during meals.

Dehydration, or thirst, may be interpreted as "I need something," resulting in you eating more. Drinking a thirst-quenching liquid prior to a meal will satisfy your thirst, and will decrease your need to drink during meals.

If you are dehydrated or your mouth is dry your saliva will be stickier (more tenacious, thicker), which may result in your first bites of food "getting stuck" when you eat. This sometimes happens to my patients in the morning. Consistently drinking prior to meals will eliminate this sticky saliva, and may help prevent the intermittent problem of the first few bites getting stuck.

Drinking during a meal may "wash" food through the small stomach, or pouch, leaving you hungry and resulting in the need to eat more in order to be satisfied.

5. Eat good-tasting, flavorful food; chew well and eat slowly.

This is very important, it is not a frivolous recommendation. There is no rule that patients cannot eat spicy, hot or tangy foods. Since you already need to eat slowly and chew for a longer time, it is easier to do so with good-tasting food that you enjoy. This is an important part of feeling satisfied after a meal.

6. Minimize high-calorie liquids and high-fat snacks.

High-calorie liquids include fruit juice, commercial smoothies, alcohol as well as cream-based soups (cream of mushroom, etc. as opposed to broth-based soups like vegetable beef). High-fat snacks include things like fried foods, potato chips, French fries.

7. Eat highly processed grain products in very small quantities, if at all.

These foods are simply not necessary for you to live a healthy life, and they are converted to sugar rapidly in your body. The result is that they affect your hunger, your weight and your health in the same way that sugar does. Highly processed grain products, such as instant oatmeal, processed breads, most pastas, tortillas and pretzels fall into this category.

8. Carbonated beverages will sometimes cause increased gas and bloating.

Carbonation typically causes burping. After surgery you will likely burp less easily and the gas will remain in your intestine, causing bloating and a "gassy feeling." Plus, if the gas isn't absorbed, it will need to pass out of your system, and if you don't burp…well, just don't guzzle two Diet Cokes on your way to the cocktail party.

9. Exercise at least five times per week

Many people do not realize that exercise is an essential part of nutrition. Not only does exercise burn calories during the activity, but it builds muscle mass that burns calories even during rest and sleep. Healthy muscle also helps balance your blood sugar and hormone levels and will help minimize cravings. Muscle toning is a critical part of obtaining successful weight loss.

Remember, if you are not sweating, you are not exercising.

10. Always take the daily nutritional supplementation that you agreed to take prior to surgery.

You asked the surgeon to perform your surgery, and you made a commitment to do your part to improve your fitness and your health. Every surgical weight-management program recommends lifelong nutritional supplementation, and all patients agree to comply with those recommendations. This is not a game, so don't treat it as one. Surgical programs are dependent on your honesty when it comes to nutritional intake.

Q Tips
Some Pointers from Doctor Q

1. Pregnancy

- It is unsafe to get pregnant during the period of rapid weight loss after bariatric surgery.

- Women may have a significant increase in fertility after bariatric surgery. This can mean that women who have previously suffered from infertility will suddenly become fertile. It is important to use birth control measures to avoid pregnancy until you have lost weight and your weight has stabilized after surgery.

- Pregnancy when you're at a healthier weight will be safer for both the mother and for the unborn baby. However, women should be seen by a doctor who understands bariatric surgery, and have your nutritional status checked if you are pregnant or plan to become pregnant. Nutritional supplementation is strongly advised, but always consult your doctor.

2. Alcohol

- Drinking alcohol is more dangerous after Gastric Bypass and Gastric Sleeve, so be careful.

- The normal stomach breaks down alcohol. After Gastric Bypass or Gastric Sleeve your stomach will not break down alcohol effectively and this will result in increased absorption of alcohol.

- Your blood alcohol level will increase faster, and remain high for longer, after bariatric surgery. This can be dangerous, causing increased brain damage and liver damage, and could also lead to the development of alcoholism.

- Alcohol also contains a lot of calories, similar to drinking a sugary soft drink.
- I recommend that patients drink minimal alcohol after bariatric surgery.

3. Drink one glass of water, or calorie-free beverage, 15-30 minutes prior to all meals.

- This does not necessarily include snacks.
- There is no reason to avoid drinking for one hour before or after meals.
- The main purpose of drinking 15-30 minutes prior to a meal is to make sure that thick saliva (you are swallowing saliva all day long without thinking about it) is not sitting in your stomach before eating. I find that when patients do this, they stop experiencing episodes where foods they are usually able to eat get occasionally "stuck" when they swallow.
  - "Getting stuck" can occur when thick saliva acts like gunk in a drain pipe and your first or second bite of food gets stuck trying to go through. You are NOT supposed to feel like you're choking when you eat slowly and chew foods well.
- A secondary benefit of this is that you won't be thirsty when you eat your meal, which means it's much easier to not drink during the meal.
- Lastly, this will give you three glasses of water, one with each meal, to help keep you hydrated during the day.

4. Minimize drinking during meals.

- It is possible that drinking, or frequent sipping, during meals will result in increased food consumption. However, a recent study done on drinking during meals after bariatric surgery showed no effect on food intake.

- If you watch the speed-eating competitions, the competitors use drinking as a way of washing food through their stomach faster so that they can pack more food in over a short period of time. I tell my patients that mimicking the speed-eating techniques of the world speed-eating champions is probably not a good plan when trying to control your weight.

- I recommend minimizing drinking during a meal.

5. One protein supplement daily (protein drink, bar, etc.) has been shown in scientific studies to enhance weight loss after bariatric surgery. Also, for people who tend to skip meals, having a high protein nutritional supplement available may improve long-term weight control.

6. Smoking

- Many surgeons require patients to quit smoking before bariatric surgery. I do not require this. However, I warn all patients that smoking increases their surgical risks and causes serious health problems long term.

- If you are going to quit smoking prior to surgery, it is safest to do so at least three months before your surgery date. Quitting smoking immediately before surgery could increase your surgical risks (according to published studies).

- I consider obesity and smoking to be two separate health concerns. I have found that people who have trouble quitting smoking before surgery often have an easier time quitting after surgery as their health improves, their mood improves, and they are not so worried about gaining weight from quitting tobacco.

7. For people with diabetes.
- If you experience a situation when you think your blood sugar is starting to drop too low, try eating a spoonful of peanut butter, or something equivalent, rather than immediately eating sugar or some candy.
- Eating sugar will rapidly increase your blood sugar, but doing this will also result in larger swings (variations) in your blood sugar and your body's insulin production, which is counterproductive for people with diabetes.
- Peanut butter, or something with a smaller amount of sugar, some complex carbohydrates, and some fat and protein, will generally increase your blood sugar quickly enough to avoid hypoglycemia without causing excessive swings in your blood sugar.

8. Drinking with a straw is OK.
- The "rule" that you should avoid using straws is tossed around by patients, online patient forums, and many program "experts" in an attempt to sound like they're giving important advice. The FACT is that there is absolutely no science (zero) behind the rule to avoid straws.
- The justification for this advice varies from "You'll swallow too much air and that will cause pain" to "It will decrease your ability to eat protein" to "It will stretch out your pouch." None of these are true.

- If you can drink comfortably using a straw, you may do so. If you can't, then don't use a straw.

9. Chewing gum is OK.
   - Avoiding gum chewing is yet another "rule" that is repeated all over the internet for various reasons, and has also made its way into many bariatric programs' "book of rules." Justification for this usually revolves around claiming that gum chewing will cause excess air swallowing. Other reasons to avoid chewing gum have included "it will exacerbate your Irritable Bowel Syndrome" (there is no proof of this) and "it will increase your desire to eat junk food" (probably the opposite is true).
   - In fact, chewing gum has been shown to decrease the desire to eat. A study published by E. Park, et al, in *Physiology and Behavior*, 2016, reported "GUM compared to Control resulted in significant suppression of hunger, desire to eat and prospective consumption ($p<0.05$)." where GUM refers to Gum Chewing.
   - Chewing gum has also been shown in research studies to reduce anxiety. One publication is by Dr. Akiyo Sasaki-Otomaru, from Tokyo Medical and Dental University in the journal <u>Clinical Practice and Epidemiology in Mental Health</u> 7(1):133-9 August 2011. The findings in this study showed that chewing gum on a regular basis may decrease anxiety, improve mood and decrease fatigue.
   - The bottom line:
     - Chewing gum for some people could result in swallowing an uncomfortable amount of air, causing intestinal gas bloat, and these people may want to avoid gum chewing.

- Chewing gum can be a useful tool to minimize hunger for some people.
- Chewing gum excessively may have some negative consequences.
- The decision to chew gum, or not, should be made by each individual based on how he feels when he does it.

10. Carbonated beverages are OK, in moderation.
   - Yes, really, this is true.
   - Carbonated beverages have been shown to increase the hunger hormone ghrelin in people with normal stomachs, but this has not been studied in people after bariatric surgery.
   - Drinking carbonated beverages has not been shown to cause problems with bone mineral density.
   - Carbonated beverages DO NOT stretch out the gastric pouch after Gastric Bypass or the small stomach after Vertical Sleeve Gastrectomy.
   - However, the effects of a significantly increased intake of gas in your stomach or intestine *may* result in increased hunger.
   - The bottom line:
     - Drinking small amounts of carbonated beverages will not cause most people problems after bariatric surgery.
     - Drinking a lot of carbonation might possibly increase your appetite.
     - Drinking a lot of carbonation may cause uncomfortable gas bloat and result in more belching (burping) and the need to pass more gas (fart).
     - Due to the increased burping and farting, I tell my patients, "Please don't drink a couple of Diet Cokes on your way to a party at my house."

11. Picture yourself at your goal weight, your Best Weight, and imagine that you *are* that person. Imagine what that person eats on a daily basis in order to maintain his or her goal weight, what exercises does that person do in order to maintain his fitness, how does that person live on a daily basis? Use this image of yourself as the goal. It is a helpful way to get in touch with what you are truly trying to achieve.

12. Remember, this book is about using bariatric surgery to achieve weight loss and long-term weight control. It's not a book specifically about living longer or eating in a way to control disease processes such as high cholesterol. You will achieve numerous health benefits from achieving a healthier weight, and controlling your weight long term. However, once you've achieved a healthier, happier weight, you can always take it to the next level by modifying your diet in order to achieve additional health benefits. My advice is to take it one step at a time; control your weight and get fit, and once you have mastered this, think about other ways to improve your health.

Unique Protocols to Enhance Comfort, Safety and Success

Many novel techniques and new technology improve patient success. Since starting one of the first highly successful laparoscopic bariatric surgery programs in America in 1999, I have developed several unique patient treatment protocols to enhance patient safety and success. Here are described a few of these protocols.

Pre-operative Diet to Decrease Liver Size; better visibility with laparoscopic camera, safer surgery

The liver is an organ that stores extra fat, and most obese people have a large liver filled with extra fat. A large liver will limit visibility during surgery, making the operation harder to do, and adding risk. In 2001, I began using a special two-week diet prior to surgery, designed specifically to decrease the size of a patient's liver prior to surgery, improving operational visibility and safety. At that time, the primary reason for surgeons being unable to complete bariatric surgery laparoscopically was the excessive size of the patient's liver.

When I mentioned my protocol at a meeting in 2003, many surgeons laughed, but a few took notes. Within a few years, more surgeons began using this protocol, and now it's used by thousands of surgeons throughout the world. This brief diet not only decreases the size of a patient's liver, but stabilizes blood sugar and improves overall nutrition prior to surgery.

Steroid Single Injection prior to Anesthesia; decrease post-operative nausea

Nausea is a common problem after general anesthesia and especially after gastrointestinal surgery. A single dose of steroids prior to surgery was shown to decrease post-operative nausea after laparoscopic gallbladder surgery. In 2003 our surgeons began giving a single dose of the steroid dexamethasone prior to surgery. We noticed an immediate decrease in post-operative nausea, and still use the protocol today.

Continuous Heparin Infusion; minimize risk of blood clots

Blood clots, called deep venous thrombosis (DVT), can form during surgery and float into the lungs, causing a pulmonary embolism (PE). These clots can be fatal. Blood thinners, such as heparin, can be used to prevent formation of DVT during surgery, but there is a significant risk of bleeding. I use a unique method of continuous low-dose heparin to prevent DVT during surgery, while minimizing the risk of bleeding. The result has been a remarkably low incidence of DVT in this program. I learned this protocol while training at the University of Chicago, and later published the protocol in a medical journal.

Non-cutting Laparoscopic Access Ports and the Zig-Zag Technique; less post-operative pain

Laparoscopic surgeons make small incisions and operate through narrow tubes, called "access ports," which leave an opening in the abdominal muscle when removed. Many surgeons close these openings with stitches to prevent hernias, and these stitches cause pain. Instead, I use ports that don't cut the abdominal muscle, and I combine this with a zig-zag technique that I developed for placing the ports so that the muscle closes effectively on its own after removing the port. This eliminates the need for painful stitches and helps patients to recover with less pain.

These are a few of the unique techniques that I employ to maximize patient comfort, safety and success.

During my career, I ran a private practice fellowship training program to teach surgeons how to perform bariatric surgery, and I taught these and other techniques to my trainees (including Dr. Justin Braverman and Dr. Channing Chin). Innovation and continuous improvement in patient care has always been a principle that I have followed.

RECOMMENDED NUTRITIONAL SUPPLEMENTS

Nutritional Supplements are Recommended for Life for All Bariatric Surgery Patients.

Almost all patients presenting for bariatric surgery evaluation already have malnutrition. Whether the risk of malnutrition after surgery is due to poor eating habits, decreased absorption of certain nutrients, or some other cause, all bariatric surgery patients are considered to be at risk for malnutrition and life-long supplementation is recommended.

After bariatric surgery, most people eat far less food which saves money, and avoiding fast food saves additional expense. These savings make weight loss surgery a money-saving procedure. The dollars saved should easily cover the cost of supplements.

We recommend only Bariatric Advantage nutritional supplements. After careful review of this company's supplement line we believe they are the best supplements. Cheap brands of vitamins typically have low amounts or poorly absorbed formulas. Patients may choose to take a different brand, but we will not comment on the quality of any other brand.

Recommended supplement regimen (modified based on lab testing)
- Daily Multivitamin
- Daily Calcium citrate
- Daily Vitamin D 5,000 IU (units)
- Daily B-Complex Supplement
- Iron supplement (100mg elemental iron)

LAB STUDIES RECOMMENDED

All Bariatric Surgery Patients at 6 and 12 Months after Surgery, and then Annually

Metabolic Panel:		
	Iron	Vitamin B1-whole blood (Thiamine)
CMP	TIBC	Vitamin B2-whole blood (Riboflavin)
CBC	Ferritin	Vitamin B3 (Nicotinamide)
PTH intact	Zinc	Vitamin B6 –plasma (pyridoxal phos)
Calcium-ionized	Folate-RBC	Vitamin B12-(Cyanocobalamin)
HgA1c	Selenium	Vitamin D3 (25-Hydroxy)
Lipid Profile	Magnesium	Vitamin E –serum (alpha tocopherol)
TSH	Phosphate	Total Testosterone (men only)

THE THREE MOST OFTEN PERFORMED BARIATRIC PROCEDURES

General Comments on the Gastric Sleeve, Gastric Bypass and Gastric Band

1. All bariatric operations are complex. The surgeon needs to perform the operation in a way that results, in the end, in very specific anatomy. In other words, if the anatomy of the stomach and intestine is not correct at the end of the operation, the operation will not work. This is not always easy to do since every person is shaped differently inside (just like we all are shaped differently on the outside). The surgeon must be focused on performing the operation correctly in order to give his or her patients the best chance for success.

2. If you eat high-calorie soft foods, or high-calorie liquids, you will be able to take in a lot of calories without feeling full. This is a way to minimize the beneficial effects of the Gastric Sleeve, the Gastric Band and the Gastric Bypass. I call this "SABOTAGE" because it means that you've chosen to undergo an operation to help you eat slowly and modify your eating pattern, and then you've figured out how to "get around" the operation. Most patients do not sabotage themselves, and as a result, they succeed in modifying their diet and losing a substantial amount of weight.

3. The speed of the operation is not a main goal; although novice surgeons may think that speed makes them "better" this is NOT TRUE. The important goal with these operations (and all surgery) is to get the operation done correctly, and to have a low complication rate. Nothing else is important. Bariatric surgeons must focus on getting the operation done correctly, and in the safest way possible.

Gastric Sleeve

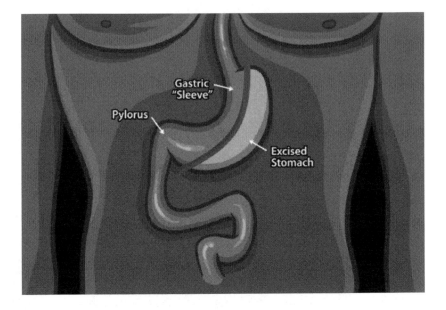

The Gastric Sleeve is simple in design. Essentially, it is a true "stomach shrinking" operation.

With the Gastric Sleeve operation, approximately 40% to 60% of the stomach is removed. However, due to the geometry involved, the *volume* of food that the stomach is able to hold is decreased by approximately 70-80%.

The upper 2/3 of the stomach is re-formed to be very narrow, with an inside diameter of between 11 to 15 mm (1/2 inch, or so). This results in a narrow stomach tube, or "sleeve" configuration. The upper part of the stomach must be narrow, and the lower part of the stomach cannot be kinked or narrowed excessively. The lowest part of the stomach, the pylorus, is a muscular area that regulates the flow of food out of the stomach and into the intestine. The pylorus, and approximately two inches of stomach before the pylorus, is left completely in place.

In order for food to pass comfortably through the stomach it must be chewed well. If you don't chew, the food will "back up" and feel uncomfortable; it may even feel as if you're choking and need to vomit. This is no different than when a person with a normal-sized stomach swallows an unchewed piece of food and it feels like it "gets stuck in their throat." Since it only takes a small amount of food to fill the new stomach, or sleeve, a person will feel like he has eaten more food. This feeling of early fullness is very useful in modifying diet and losing weight.

Gastric Bypass

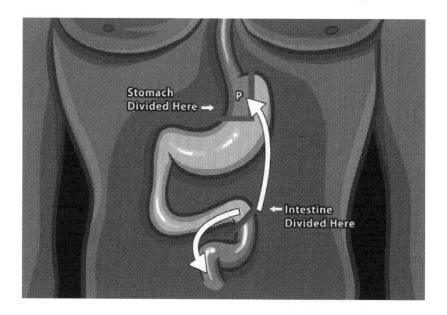

For the Gastric Bypass, the stomach and intestine are cut in the manner shown in Diagram #1, above.

The lower part of the intestine (darker colored in the diagram) is moved up and attached to the small upper portion of the stomach, labeled "P" for pouch.

In the body this move is only four or five inches, as these organs lie very close together inside our abdomen.

The upper portion of the intestine is reattached to the lower portion of the intestine approximately 100cm downstream from where it was originally attached.

There is roughly 400cm (12 feet) of small intestine, and 200cm (6 feet) of large intestine in our bodies. All of this intestine is within our abdominal cavity, curled around itself in an organized way so that it rarely gets tangled up. When surgeons do cancer operations, they routinely cut out a section of intestine, and then attach the two cut ends back together. A similar technique is used to reattach the stomach and intestine for the gastric bypass.

As you can see above, a gastric bypass results in bypassing most of the stomach, and a short portion of the intestine.

The stomach functions mainly to grind up, dissolve, and digest the food we eat.

Most nutrition is absorbed in the intestine, all 400 cm of it, and some nutrition is absorbed in the large intestine. Very little nutrition is absorbed in the stomach.

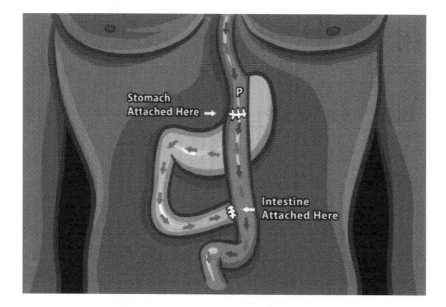

In Diagram #2, you can see the stomach and intestine reattached in final form.

Food goes first into the small stomach, called a pouch, "P," and then travels immediately into the intestine where absorption of nutrition takes place.

Since the small stomach pouch cannot do a very good job of grinding up, dissolving and digesting food, patients with this operation must chew food well. The enzymes people have in their mouth are extremely effective at digesting food, so adequate chewing will improve nutrition.

The shaded portion of the esophagus, the stomach, and the intestine is where the food you eat travels. The blue arrows indicate food, and the green arrows show that acid and enzymes from the stomach, as well as bile from your liver, and pancreatic juices from your pancreas, all still travel through the bypassed stomach and intestine, and then mix back in with the food you have eaten. The fluids coming from your bypassed stomach and intestine, liver and pancreas are all needed for adequate digestion of nutrition. The bypassed stomach and intestine continue to live normally, making important fluids for digestion and absorption. If there is a reason to reconnect the stomach and intestine back to the original anatomy, as was present before the gastric bypass, it can be done, and food will generally go back to being digested and absorbed in the way it was before your bariatric surgery. Of course, you will very likely regain some of the weight you lost.

No organs are removed during a standard gastric bypass operation.

Dumping:

One last topic I need to discuss is the phenomenon of dumping. Dumping is very misunderstood by most patients as well as by many physicians. The fact is, dumping is a very useful effect of the gastric bypass. I call dumping an "effect" and not a "side effect" because I consider it to be one of the most useful effects of this operation.

Dumping occurs when certain types of foods, primarily food with concentrated sugar (e.g. ice cream), enters the intestine before it's been digested by the enzymes present in the stomach and first part of the intestine. Since, as you can see in the above diagram, the stomach and first part of the intestine are bypassed, the intestine that is attached to the gastric pouch will "see" the food before it mixes and digests with the enzymes coming from the pancreas and liver. When the small intestine experiences concentrated sweets before they have been properly digested, the intestine will "dump."

Dumping describes the phenomenon of the intestine reacting to a caustic substance, in this case undigested sweets or sugars, and trying to flush this caustic substance through. To flush it through it will flood itself with water and wash the contents through to the large intestine. This is often accompanied by a feeling of indigestion or cramping. The large intestine then reacts to all this fluid coming downstream too fast, and if there is too much, it will get rid of this fluid; in other words, you will have diarrhea. Remember, this occurs almost exclusively as a result of eating concentrated sweets.

I consider this a very useful phenomenon. Remember, people who undergo gastric bypass are people who have been battling obesity for years. Eating concentrated sweets is hardly a good weight-control maneuver, so experiencing adverse effects when you eat more than a couple of bites of a sugar-filled dessert is not a bad thing.

In my experience, most patients experience dumping only in the mild form. However, if a person were to eat a large amount of sugar after a gastric bypass, he could develop so much fluid in his intestine that he becomes light headed, and could faint, so in the extreme form this could be dangerous.

The only patients that I've had who complain about dumping after gastric bypass are patients that don't get it. Yes, there is individual variation in how severe dumping is after gastric bypass, with some patients experiencing severe dumping and others not getting it at all. Patients who find they do not get dumping at all have come in to me and complained; they sometimes ask, "How do I keep from eating sweets?" and I tell them they have to avoid sweets on their own.

Historically, gastric dumping existed before the gastric bypass operation. It was observed in patients that had operations for ulcers, or for cancer, where a portion of the stomach was removed, and the stomach and intestine were reconnected with the Roux-en-Y configuration seen above. Dumping also occurs, although rarely, in patients with normal anatomy. When the stomach empties its contents into the intestine too fast, the intestine can react, and dump.

Gastric Band

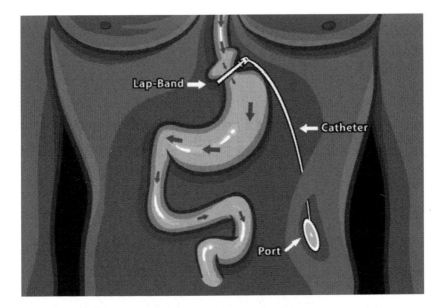

The Gastric Band is a hard, plastic device that is wrapped around the upper part of the stomach. It is attached by a thin tube, called a catheter, to a hollow reservoir in the shape of a disc. The disc-shaped reservoir has one hard side with a round metal plate and one soft side made of rubber. The entire system—reservoir (called a port), catheter, and band—is filled with saline (salt water).

When a bariatric surgeon places the band around your stomach, he connects it to the catheter and the port, placing the port below your skin but on top of your abdominal muscle. The port is positioned with the rubber side up and the metal plate down and stitched in position.

In order to tighten or loosen your band, the surgeon will pass a small needle through your skin, through the rubber side of the port, and into the reservoir. The metal plate stops him from passing the needle too far. He will then add or withdraw saline, to tighten or loosen the band, as needed.

When a person with the Gastric Band eats, food passes down the esophagus into the small stomach pouch above the band, then passes through the band and into the stomach. Because the band restricts the flow of food through the upper stomach, a person with a Gastric Band will need to chew food very well to prevent it from getting stuck. Food will stay in the upper stomach for a while, giving the person a sense of "fullness," before passing downward through the main portion of the stomach.